Thank You for purchasing this book!

**Welcome to
Dr. Lyn Is In**

How to Motivate Your Clients to Change

**For Therapists, Coaches, Teachers,
Trainers and Healthcare Professionals**

**Author, Lyn Kelley, Ph.D., CPC
Certified Professional Coach**

*"My mission is to empower people to move to the
next level of success in their lives."*

What others are saying about Dr. Lyn's Books

Lyn Kelly is AWESOME. Her e-books are the books. There are so many garbage marketing books at the bookstore, garbage marketing seminars, people trying to take a lot of money from health care practitioners teaching marketing.

Every other book/class is just psycho-babble. Full of stupid tips likes "be positive," "attract clients to yourself," "whatever you do, do consistent." OK, the psych stuff and being in the correct frame of mind of important. It's not worthless, but to be successful you also need an action plan. You need the right mindset, plus a concrete plan to execute.

Lyn Kelley does both! And she has amazing actions plans. The great things is, she has a whole list, full of details on how to execute each one. If one strategy isn't right for you, another one will work. Her e-books are the absolute best!

---Saul Marcus, Pittsburgh, PA

Thank you so much for your book. You're right, it does work as soon as you use it. Your workbook exercises were most helpful. I am already getting positive responses.

---Charie Levy, MFT Brooklyn, NY

Dear Lyn, I found your workshop so inspirational! It has taken me to another level in my consciousness about the work we do as therapists and it has further inspired me to continue my pursuits in the realm of Organizational Development and Transformation. Your being is quite a catalyst. I appreciate what you are doing very much and feel honored to have been able to experience your work and its profound effect, first-hand.

---Jeanine Gonzalez, Dallas, TX

How to Motivate Your Clients to Change
By Lyn Kelley, Ph.D., CPC
Certified Professional Coach

"Nothin' to it but to do it."
---Lyn Kelley

Table of Contents

Introduction:
Why Should You Become a Motivational
Coach/Expert?
6 Great Reasons
What does a "Motivational Coach" do?

PART ONE: **Philosphy of Motivation**

Chapter 1: **Definitions of Motivation**
Where Does Motivation Come From?
The Main Theories of What Motivates People

Chapter 2: **Assessing Healthy Goals**
How to Help Clients Set Healthy and Attainable
Goals
Achievement Motivation
Healthy Pursuit of Goals
Definitions of Success
Internal vs External Motivation
Assessment

Chapter 3: **Comparison of Professional
and Self-Help Literature**
The Best of Self Help and Pop Psychology
Comparisons and Common Threads

Differences
Positives & Negatives of Self Help and Pop
Psychology

Chapter 4: How People Change
How Top Coaches Motivate Their Clients
What Makes People Change
Pain vs Pleasure
How Quickly Can People Change?
Gradual Change
What You Can Change and What You Can't

PART TWO: Overcoming Obstacles

Chapter 5: Success Sabotage
The 7 Major Self Sabotages
How to Help Clients Move Past Their Blocks

Chapter 6: Thought and Attitude Transformation
The First and Most Important Thing to Do
Influences on Change
Developing Ambition
Controlled Focus
Cognitive Strategies for Self-Defeating Statements
Deriving Inspiration from Stories of Others who
Overcame Adversity
Using Life Traumas or Difficulties as Motivators

PART THREE. The Motivational Process

Chapter 7: Personal Vision and Mission Statement
How to Draw Out Your Clients Passions and Dreams

The 3 V's: Values, Vision and Voice
The "PPPP" Principle

Chapter 8: Goal Setting and Action Planning

The Easy "5 Step Process" of Goal Setting
Setting an Action Plan
Prioritizing
Setting Sub-Goals and Tasks
Maintenance
Termination
Relapse

Chapter 9: Social Aspects of Motivation

How to Create Social Support
Role Models
Mentors, Sponsors, Teachers, and Coaches
Partners
Fly in "V" Formation

Chapter 10: Spiritual Aspects of Motivation

Peak Experiences
Positive Affirmations and Self Reinforcement
Visualizations That Inspire Clients to Amazing Growth
Your Words are Your Power

PART FOUR: Implementation

Chapter 11: Keeping Clients in Coaching Until Goals are Achieved

Hidden Reasons Clients End Programs Too Soon
How to Keep Clients in Their Programs and Remain Motivated

3 Things to Give Clients Before They Leave Their Session
Reactivating Former Clients
Program Structure
Program Goals
Program Support
The Best Motivational Strategies
Ending a Coaching Program

Chapter 12: Motivation for the Coach and/or Helping Professional
How to Keep Yourself Motivated
Preventing Caregiver Burnout
Operating at Peak Performance
The 7-Step Success Cycle

Bibliography

Introduction

Coaching is a conversation, a dialogue, whereby the coach and the individual interact in a dynamic exchange to achieve goals, enhance performance and move the individual forward to greater success.
---Zeus and Skiffington

Yes, people can change! People can change even if they don't want to. There are specific strategies to help people change. This book will give you these strategies. I've spent the past 30 years researching motivation and change, and I will give you the BEST of the BEST ideas that have been proven to work. These strategies are true, tested, and trusted by the majority of experts. You don't have to read all the books and research articles – I've already done that for you. This book will provide a synopsis of what has been proven to work for the majority of people over time.

The primary goal of any helping intervention is to create change. Change is difficult for most people however, and clients need to be sufficiently motivated to create and sustain desired changes. The aim of this book is to address those problems and suggest ways for coaches to overcome them: to become motivational experts and have the ability to implement successful, organized coaching or motivational programs with their clients.

Throughout this book I will refer to any motivational practitioner as "coach." Anyone can be a coach. Anyone working with children or teens should learn how to coach. Anyone who consults or advises people should learn how to coach. If you are a healthcare or mental health provider, it is very important that you understand the theory of coaching and behavior change, because your primary goal is to cause your clients to change their behaviors for the good of their overall health. All of these principles can be applied to anyone who wants to help people change for the better. The term "treatment" or "program" will be used for anyone who is currently under the care or guidance of a coach or healthcare provider.

<u>**Six Great Reasons to Become a Motivational Coach or Expert**</u>

Why should you become a coach or motivational expert? There are many reasons. The <u>first</u> and most important reason is that when you know what motivates people, your clients will gain successes that <u>they otherwise might never have been able to</u>. Why should a client hire <u>you</u> as their coach, when there is an over-abundance of coaches in almost every city? If you can show that you have expertise in motivating client change, you will stand out over coaches with traditional training. <u>Second</u>, if you are looking to increase your fee-for-service clientele, you will need to attract a more affluent, personal growth oriented market. As the socio-economic climate of our society increases, so does the desire for personal, business and career coaches. Motivational coaching is the wave of the future, so it is a great niche to specialize in and to use to build your practice.

<u>Third</u>, the public has been inundated over the past 20 years with self-help books on motivation, a trend which directly influences the therapy, coaching and healthcare professions. The plethora of self-help books raises the question of whether people will still seek out professional assistance when aisles of self-help books beckon from the corner bookstore. Coaches and therapists provide crucial functions that self-help books cannot, but given the popularity of self-help literature, it seems wise for coaches to use

the self-help trend to their <u>advantage</u> rather than ignore it.

Coaching provides a framework in which ideas that clients discover in self-help books can be tested and synthesized with other issues raised in a more personal context. Moreover, coaching gives clients a forum to address contradictions and inconsistencies that they discover in self-help material. It is useful for coaches to regard self-help books as a catalyst that encourages clients to be introspective, think psychologically, and seek out therapy and/or coaching. Accordingly, if coaches can learn the basic premises of the self-help movement and incorporate them into treatment with interested clients, they can use the proliferation of self-help books as a selling point, a way to increase their practices rather than a threat to them. My intention in this book is to include the best and most relevant aspects of both self-help and professional literature about motivation and to apply the material to a clinical setting.

<u>Fourth</u>, becoming a motivational expert can greatly assist you with the major problem in getting clients to become consistently motivated -- <u>resistance</u>. Often, it is tempting to label a client's behavior as resistance when in fact the issue is a lack of knowledge or skill, a long-standing fear, self-doubts about competency, the practice of self-sabotage, or a pervasive lack of self-esteem. Even if clients do not suffer from any of these concerns, they may not know how to approach a goal and formulate an action plan for accomplishing it. In this case, what the clients lack is external: a teacher, guide, or coach to assist them in organizing and undertaking the pursuit of their goals. Coaches who are trained in the subject of motivation can help their clients formulate goals, overcome resistance, and develop the necessary confidence and skill to succeed.

Because of their regular contact with clients, coaches are ideally situated to act as motivational guides.

The <u>fifth</u> reason to become a motivational expert is to learn how you can help clients to remain in their program until they are have achieved their goals. Research shows that at least 45% of clients leave treatment too soon. This problem -- <u>client loss</u> -- is probably the greatest, yet least talked about problem in the helping professions. Loss of clientele, loss of referrals, and loss of income all lead to loss of self-esteem and income for the coach. Becoming an expert in the field of motivation and successfully helping clients become motivated will work to motivate the coach as well. This book is full of suggestions for ways to get your clients motivated and then get them to stay in treatment until their treatment goals have been achieved.

And finally, a <u>sixth</u> reason to become a motivational expert is that it is <u>good for you, the coach</u>. When your clients meet their goals, turn their lives around, achieve lasting positive change, it leads to your feelings of professional self confidence and self fulfillment. Chapter Twelve on self-motivation addresses in more detail the relevance of the subject to coaches themselves and suggests ways that coaches can regain motivation in their own lives and practices.

<u>What Does a Motivational Coach Do?</u>

The definition of coaching is *helping people with goal achievement*. The definition of motivation is *the desire to move*. As a motivational coach, you help people pull up their own desires to move forward toward their goals. According to James Prochaska (2005) there are over 400 therapeutic modalities being used by counselors today. Coaching is simply ONE of those modalities. Anyone can call themselves a coach, however, one must be able to show <u>competency</u> in coaching before stating he/she provides this service. Counselors trained in coaching can move in and out of the coaching modality during therapeutic treatment. Throughout this book I interchange the terms "coaching" and "therapy," so keep in mind that coaching is a therapeutic technique. In this book I will refer to "the motivator" as a *coach* and "the motivatee" as a *client*.

The goal of this book is to give human service providers new ideas about ways in which to help their clients make positive personal change. The focus in coaching is to move clients forward, however, at times clients will become "stuck" and therefore it is helpful to have some motivational strategies to assist them in becoming "un-stuck." Becoming a specialist in the field of motivation and/or coaching is a great way to build your practice and income while helping others.

The best coaches really care about people. They have a sincere interest in people.
---Byron & Catherine Pulsifer, from *What Are People's Expectations of a Coach?*

Chapter One:
Definitions of Motivation

A good coach will make his players see what they can be rather than what they are.
---Ara Parasheghian

The word motivation is derived from the Latin word "movere," meaning, to move. Thus to motivate someone is to incite motion. Motivation is brought about by having a motive, a drive or impulse that causes one to act. Coaches can help their clients gain motivation through helping them define their motives. Accordingly, it is useful for coaches to think of themselves as motivators.

Where Does Motivation Come From?

Motivation, like any other personal characteristic, comes from genetics, environment, and experience. Motivation occurs in a large variety of forms and contexts. The term is widely used, from the classic teacher's comment on a report card that the student is bright but "lacks motivation" to the now seemingly omnipresent "motivational speakers" who give workshops and appear on Oprah. Within the field of psychology, motivation is divided into categories -- it can be geared toward power, toward affiliation, toward aggression, and toward achievement. It can be sudden--an internal surge of passion, or it can be adopted more slowly and grudgingly, because of the knowledge that one should improve something about one's life, even if one doesn't really want to do the work that is involved.

The Main Theories of What Motivates People

Self help books focus on "achievement motivation" which can be defined as a desire for significant accomplishment. Motivation can be defined in different terms according to different psychological theories. Some of these theories are described in brief here.

Psychoanalytically, motivation represents the pursuit to fulfill repressed needs and drives. Freud contributed greatly to the field of motivational change, by defining his "Pleasure Principle." He believed that human psychology is governed by the tendency to seek pleasure and avoid pain. Jung's motivational theory is based on consciousness-raising -- the individual's innate need to uncover the "self" -- one's true, authentic being.

From a behavioral standpoint, motivation is defined as creating a change in behavior and is expressed in terms of physical drives: desires and needs. B.F. Skinner's major premise was, "we do what we do because of what happens to us when we do it."

Humanistically, it entails the journey toward self-actualization. Abraham Maslow believed that, as their lower level needs were met, people would continually move up the "hierarchy of needs" ladder toward self-actualization. The goal of self-actualization is that of reaching a state in which one feels fulfilled in life and can live in the present moment.

Existential theory discusses motivation in terms of the person's innate need for meaning. Alfred Adler believed that all our drives have a purpose -- to feel important -- to move us from a feeling of minus to a feeling of plus.

<u>Scientific</u> theory focuses more on intrinsic motivation, and defines it in terms of innate curiosity.

The <u>social or systemic</u> element of motivation can be defined in relation to environmental pressures, to the surrounding people who exert influence and thus define the terms of motivation. Adler felt strongly that people could not be studied in isolation, but only in terms of social context. We are motivated by the effect we will have on others.

<u>Cognitive-behavioral</u> theory states that the primary factors that contribute to achievement motivation are self-determination or autonomy (feeling in control of one's situation rather than controlled by external agents) and a sense of competence (self-perception of ability). In several studies, Bandura tested the role of self-efficacy as it related to motivation and demonstrated that an individual's <u>belief</u> about his or her ability to accomplish an activity directly affected performance. Cognitive restructuring has proven to be very beneficial to the motivational process, and will be explained more fully in later chapters.

New Thought theory is more spiritual in nature. There is a spiritual revolution going on in the world today, and more and more people are becoming motivated by their spiritual and religious beliefs. On of the most popular new thought ideas is that of "quantum physics," or "quantum energy." The book/movie *The Secret* exemplifies this concept. The premise of *The Secret* is the "law of attraction," that is, "like attracts like," and "thoughts become things."

As you can see, we have an abundance of theories from the most respected contributors to the field of psychology and change. Each of these theories has legitimacy, and it is possible to support many or all of them. This book utilizes an integrated approach. As I explain in Chapter Three, all self help literature has its basis in at least one of these preceding theories. While these were the predominate theories in my research, there are many more.

*You get the best effort from others not by lighting a fire beneath them,
but by building a fire within.*
---Bob Nelson

Chapter Two:
Assessing Healthy and Unhealthy Goals

Every man is the architect of his own fortune.
---Sallust

Achievement Motivation

Abraham Maslow, the great humanistic psychologist, said there are two types of motivation, deficiency motivation and growth motivation. Deficiency motivation is the desire to fill a perceived void in one's life, particularly a basic need such as food, water, air, shelter, or warmth. Growth motivation is the desire to improve one's life, after all the basic needs and comforts have been met.

This book focuses predominantly on achievement motivation, since in many ways it is the most relevant to work with clients who want to change something about their lives and are having difficulty doing so. With respect to achievement motivation, there are still several elements to keep in mind. One, which will be discussed later, is the difference between intrinsic and extrinsic motivation -- namely, whether one is motivated because of an inherent curiosity and desire for knowledge or productivity, or because of pressures exerted from the outside, such as from teachers, employers, and family members. Another issue is that there are several phases of motivation. These are: 1) having a goal to which one aspires, 2) implementing a course of action that leads toward that goal, 3) persisting in one's quest of the goal over a period of time and in the face of difficulties and, 4) achieving the goal successfully. All of these phases need to be considered when assessing the whole process of motivation.

A debate in *American Psychologist* exemplifies this principle. Carol Sansone and Judith Harackiewicz chastise the author of a previous article for "summariz[ing] the effects of rewards on intrinsic motivation solely in terms of their outcomes." Rather, they argue, "one must examine the process in addition to the outcome" in order for the results of the study to be valid.

Healthy Pursuit of Goals

Before a coach recommends that clients "go for their goals," "do it now," "make it happen," it is important to assess the clients' goals. <u>First</u>, many clients begin treatment with <u>goal conflict</u>. Clients may not even realize they have goal conflict -- they are either trying to achieve too much at once, or they want too many different things and cannot start any one thing due to their confusion. It is important for the coach to assist the client in sifting through the "muck" and determining what it is the client really wants, and what it is that the client can actually do at this time toward attaining it.

<u>Second</u>, the goal may not be a healthy one. Healthy goals are those that take into account the pursuant's well-being, in addition to the well-being of others. If clients state that they desire something that is dangerous to themselves or to society, it is the coach's responsibility to assess their seriousness, determine whether outside intervention is needed, and to deter them from these goals and help them develop more positive goals. For example, if a client's goal is to get revenge on his ex-boss who fired him unfairly, the clinician must attempt to assist the client in the healing process before discussing future goals. If the client is rebounding from a painful experience, it is important to work through that experience before focusing on goals that stem from the residual pain. If the client's goal is to "beat

the competition" in a particular business, it is possible that the underlying motivation is again one of revenge, which of course is unhealthy.

Another example of unhealthy goals occurs in the case of clients suffering from a type of <u>self-defeating personality disorder</u>. They may be motivated to pursue jobs or relationships, but the jobs and relationships that they pursue will be destructive to their well-being and in the end will hinder rather than further their aims. The unhealthy goal should be stated as such by the coach and directly confronted as one which the coach refuses to support or join with. Not only is the urge for revenge or the arrangement of self-defeat unhealthy, but it fails to address the underlying problems. In psychoanalytic terms, it is a manifestation of a repetition compulsion that stems from a repressed trauma that has not yet been addressed. For example viewing others as victimizers often stems from an earlier, unrelated experience of victimization. Therefore, the first thing the coach should do in broaching the motivational process is to explore and uncover the client's underlying motives for the goal and discuss them with the client in order to determine whether the client's goal is a healthy one that should be pursued.

The <u>third</u> element that coaches should address is <u>overall health</u>, by looking at clients' goals within a holistic framework. As coaches, we need to be very careful that we do not assume that clients are healthy just because they are functioning well in particular areas (in fact, high-functioning people are sometimes the most unhealthy because their problems are so successfully masked). Thus, we should explore all areas of our clients lives for problems and encourage health and balance in mental, physical, emotional, spiritual, interpersonal, and professional areas. Realistic and healthy goals will complement the rest of an individual's lifestyle, will mesh with the individual's other goals, and will therefore serve to build self-esteem. Ways in which coaches can assist their clients in a healthy planning and action process toward achievement of their goals are discussed throughout this book.

Specific goals must correlate with a person's interests, value system, and life-goals in order to be meaningful to that individual. For the individual to be optimally motivated, the goals should correspond to his or her level of expertise and be able to be completed in a manageable time frame. Unlike a wish or fantasy, a goal must be attainable. Thus, for an individual who began playing the violin at age 30, playing in a string quartet at a friend's marriage is a more realistic goal than becoming concert master of the Berlin Philharmonic. In general, more difficult goals elicit higher motivation, but this is contingent both on the person's confidence about his or her ability to complete the task and on the goal being challenging without being unreasonably difficult. Moreover, the more attractive the goal to the individual, the better his or her performance is likely to be, so it is important that the goal selected is one that the individual really cares about.

Some motivational experts propound the idea of focusing single-mindedly on one goal, to the exclusion of everything else, yet there is an element of danger in prescribing such a path. We have all heard stories of people who have done this, first becoming extremely successful in a particular field and then "bombing." These people may end their success by overdosing on drugs or alcohol, they may suffer a heart attack or other serious health problem, they may commit a crime for which they must serve most of their remaining life in prison, or they may even commit suicide. This scenario is so common that it deserves attention, particularly for the mental health clinician.

There are pros and cons to setting one goal and pursuing it fervently. Some people believe that an obsessive approach is the only way to realize one's dreams. According to this philosophy, everything that one gives up in the process of pursuing this one goal was predominantly a distraction and thus better-off gone. Alternatively, some people believe that the ideal is to have a balanced life, and that obsessive, single-minded motivation is as much of a problem as no motivation at all. One factor to keep in mind is a time frame. If the goal is a short-term one, such as during the next week or month, then the obsessive approach might not be harmful, since many of the aspects of life that one neglects for this week can probably be attended to the subsequent week. However, if the goal is a long term one -- before I die, I want to -- then the obsessive approach becomes more problematic. The dilemma is exemplified in the case of top athletes, who sacrifice everything to train in their sport. The single-minded focus pays off when they make it to the Olympics and perhaps even win a medal. However, the dangers of this narrow focus are revealed when the Olympics are over. Many athletes have attested to undergoing periods of severe depression after retiring from their sport. Because they have neglected academics, family, friends, and hobbies, they are suddenly confronted with a void and question their ability to pursue a new and unrelated goal of perhaps a less overwhelming nature. The other danger of pursuing one goal to the exclusion of all others is that one's whole sense of self rests on this one success. Should one fail, or even perform only at a mediocre level, it is easy to internalize this assessment as one that reflects on one's whole character rather than merely this one activity. In *Life's Too Short!*, Abraham Twerski writes, "The goal of changing the self-concept [of a narrowly-focused overachiever] to a positive one is not to convert an ambitious person into a beachcomber, but to allow the person to perform at the same level without jeopardizing his or her physical and emotional health."

As I pointed out in Chapter One, Bandura's tests demonstrated that if a person believes that he/she is capable of succeeding at something, he/she has a much greater chance of performing well at that activity or task. Thus, ability is not fixed but depends on self-perception. Moreover, a sense of self-efficacy can be fostered by setting attainable goals -- ones that are neither too large nor too distant. In his study, Deci defined such goals as "optimally challenging." Success on these small goals fosters a greater intrinsic motivation for related activities, and can thus eventually lead to the achievement of larger goals for which the smaller ones were stepping stones.

An important element of pursuing one's goals is the ability to modify one's behavior and adapt to changing circumstances. A successful statistician, who has written statistics texts throughout his adult life, has now begun at age 80 to write a history of statistics. He feels that he is no longer able to stay on the cutting edge of research but that his many years in the field give him an advantage when he turns to the history of statistics. A crucial function of the coach is to act as a guide for your clients -- to help them assess whether their goals are realistic or whether they need to be modified or adapted.

Definitions of Success

Success can be defined in a number of ways, depending on who is defining it, his or her perspective, and the type of activity being evaluated. Success for a student who is math-phobic may mean passing calculus and never having to take another math class, whereas success for a student who excels in math and hopes to attend MIT may mean getting an A+ in the same calculus course. Success can be defined according to external and internal criteria. It is important for the coach to discuss with clients the clients' definitions of success and perhaps encourage them to broaden these definitions to include more attainable goals and standards.

External criteria are factors such as material wealth and the perceptions of others. In this regard, success might mean earning more than $100,000 dollars a year or receiving an award as Outstanding Teacher of the Year. External criteria are mediated by cultural contexts and influences: success may be defined very differently in Kenyan culture and Thai culture -- or even in the cultures of Northern California and Southern California. Internally-defined criteria consist of one's own perceptions and definitions of success, based on a sense of self-efficacy and volition: a sense of control over the task and of success as defined by knowledge and skills acquired. Internal criteria may also consist of satisfaction of goal fulfillment, a feeling of accomplishment and a sense of meaning in one's purpose in life.

Internal vs. External Motivation

In studies of extrinsic motivation, the participants' interest and motivation to repeat or continue with an activity wane after they have received a reward for doing well, because the activity has become externally controlled and success is dependent on the reward. The concept of intrinsic motivation, which rests on a belief in the innate psychological desire to be competent and autonomous, arose during the 1950's in response to the exclusive focus on extrinsic motivation of the learning and drive theorists. This paralleled a general increase in interest in individual capabilities for development and change that developed in large part in reaction to the fascism and exertion of control that characterized the horrors of the Nazi era (Seligman, *What You Can Change and What You Can't*). The truly novel nature of the contemporary belief in intrinsic motivation and the capacity of the individual to will and to bring about self change is detailed in Seligman's book. He contrasts this current belief with the enduring historical belief that one's role is determined by class, gender, family profession, God's will, etc. -- an outlook that disregards individual character and self-determination.

Nonetheless, there is still a wide range of attitudes toward the power of self-determination. It is useful for coaches to find out where their clients stand on the self-determination spectrum: some may be waiting for divine intervention to solve their problems, while others may think they have absolute control. The optimal goal is of course a healthy combination that rests on gaining insight into what can genuinely be controlled by the individual and what cannot. Once this is understood, the client can concentrate his or her energy on developing attainable goals. Interestingly, this balance is reflected in the recitation used by Alcoholics Anonymous: *"God grant me the serenity to accept the things I cannot change, the courage to change the things I can, and the wisdom to know the difference."* The saying combines the belief in a higher power with the belief in self-determination. The centrality of this combination to the 12-step philosophy is perhaps a partial explanation for the organization's astounding popularity and endurance.

The question of whether internal or external motivation produces more effective and/or longer lasting results is the subject of ongoing debate, and many theorists are now stressing the interrelation of the two types. Jung's work focuses on integration of both the "ego" (external) and the "self" (internal). Also, it has been shown that as one pursues a goal for extrinsic reasons, the motivation often transfers into intrinsic needs. Thus, what starts out simply as a desire for a material thing, can evolve, over the course of time, into a part of the person's being, or core self.

<u>Assessment</u>

In summary, the main points to assess in determining healthiness of client's goals are:

--How one feels about him/herself in relation to self, others, <u>and</u> environment during the pursuit, attainment, and post-attainment of goals
--Goals are congruent with the client's core values, and are prioritized yet flexible
--Take into account the client's well-being, as well as the well-being of others, and of society
--Take into account the client's "underlying motives"
--"Optimally challenging" -- realistic -- attainable -- neither too easy or too difficult
--Holistic framework and overall health of the client during pursuit of goals

Be like a postage stamp. Stick to one thing until you get there.
---Josh Billings

Move toward that which makes you feel good and be happy.
---Wayne Dyer

Comparison and Common Threads

Since most clients who enter a program are reading self-help books, it seems important that mental health professionals have a sense of what these books are about so that they can respond to their clients in an informed manner. Most self-help and pop psychology literature stems from the primary psychological theories in professional literature. For example, Tony Robbins read over 700 books and studied the work of many prominent psychological theorists before writing his first best-seller, *Unlimited Power*. Likewise, Wayne Dyer asserts that the person who most influenced his work was Abraham Maslow. And, exemplifying an even more direct impact, Gail Sheehy's successful book *Passages* is a popularization of Daniel Levinson's study of adult development, *The Seasons of a Man's Life*.

There are a surprising number of commonalties in the approaches to motivation expressed in popular and professional literature. For example, the self-help best-seller *Do It! Let's Get Off Our Buts* begins "There's a lot of good news about our dreams: By pursuing any *one* of our dreams, we can find fulfillment. We don't need to pursue them all." The sentiment is a rephrasing of the theory of optimal motivation -- namely, motivation and performance are higher if there are neither too few nor too many goals. Tests have shown that too few goals leads to under-motivation and too many goals leads to being overwhelmed and thus performing less well (Costanza, Woody, and Slater in *Achievement and Motivation*).

One of the main subjects that self-help literature shares with professional literature is that of intrinsic motivation. Professional studies have shown that intrinsic motivation leads to higher performance and more enduring motivation than extrinsic motivation, which depends on external rewards or punishments. This focus on the innate ability of the individual to effect change and realize his or her particular dreams is the central tenet of self-help literature. It is expressed in the title of one of the chapters of *Do It! Let's Get Off Our Buts*: "Programmed for failure but built for success." The implication is that even when all external forces conspire to frustrate one's success, there is an internal ability and power that can overcome these forces -- that intrinsic motivation can lead to success no matter what the external circumstances. This phrasing is an overstatement that ignores the interjection of external influences, but it nonetheless reflects an unwavering commitment to the powers of intrinsic motivation. The popularity of the book accentuates how eager American society is to accept this model of motivation and personal control. However, the belief is far from universal: it is a product of American history and cultural values, and it is important for coaches to keep this cultural element in mind when working with clients from varied cultural and religious backgrounds.

Because of my belief in the importance of recognizing the influence of popular psychology and self-help literature on contemporary American culture and on people's beliefs about psychology, I endeavor to integrate references to popular texts as well as professional ones into this book.

Differences

The problem with most of the self-help advocates is that they rely predominantly on their own opinions, single case histories, and testimonials, such as before and after snapshots of a person who lost weight. Outcome studies in professional research are the best evidence of what really works. Case histories (while enjoyable reading) are unreliable as a source of general patterns and rules of behavior, because they are isolated instances. Authors' opinions are also unreliable when they are not backed by the results of outcome studies.

Some of the positive aims of pop psychology books are to build readers' self-confidence, to help them overcome a sense of worthlessness, doubt, or failure, and thereby to help foster a sense of capability and competence that will lead to intrinsic motivation. And one of the most useful aspects of the popular books on motivation is that they often provide a <u>structure</u> for making changes that clinical books do not. Because these books are written so that readers are able to apply the ideas to their own lives, they tend to emphasize <u>practical strategies</u> for developing goals and becoming organized in one's pursuit of change. For example, many self-help books offer useful exercises for articulating one's goals, breaking them down into attainable sub-goals, and overcoming one's inertia and getting started on a program of action. If their clients are interested in self-help books, coaches can incorporate this element into the process as a way of helping their clients develop a plan for achieving their goals.

The down side of these popular books is that they tend to generalize extravagantly so as to make their advice applicable to all readers. Also, in their endeavor to foster a sense of empowerment in the reader, they tend to overemphasize what the individual can accomplish. One book suggests that the reader create an imaginary sanctuary where he or she can retreat when the going gets rough; it then goes on to suggest that the reader include in this sanctuary a Master Teacher with whom to confer when feeling doubtful about a course of action or about the ability to succeed -- a suggestion which dangerously ignores the situations in which a real expert needs to be consulted. Furthermore, self-help books tend to exaggerate how quickly change can be accomplished and goals can be met. When change is wrought instantaneously, without the accompaniment of insight, processing, and maintenance, the triumph is usually fleeting, the change temporary.

<u>Positives & Negatives of Self Help and Pop Psychology</u>

In summary, some of the more <u>positive</u> aspects of self help literature are:

--Convenience and availability
--Easy to understand - usually written more for the concrete learner
--Practical and useful
--Provides structure
--Builds readers' self confidence
--Some of the more <u>negative</u> aspects of self help literature are:
--Provide little or no empirical data
--Little or no back-up research for theories and opinions presented
--Tends to generalize -- makes advice applicable to all readers
--Tends to overemphasize what an individual can accomplish
--Tends to exaggerate how quickly change can be accomplished

How am I going to live today in order to create the tomorrow I'm committed to?
---Tony Robbins

People underestimate their capacity for change.
There is never a right time to do a difficult thing.
---John Porter

What Makes People Change?

As I have discussed earlier, there are a variety of factors and forces that can cause a person to create self change. There are internal forces, as well as external forces. People change to avoid pain and/or to seek pleasure. People can change from a single thought, emotion, catharsis, event, idea, statement, experience or decision. Sometimes people change because they want to, sometimes they change because they have to.

Pain and Pleasure

The motivation for any change is <u>to make one's life better</u>. As Freud's pleasure principle states, human psychology is governed by the tendency to seek pleasure and avoid pain. If a person perceives making a change as positive, one that will improve the quality of life and bring about feelings of pleasure, this will begin to provide the motivation to make the change. If, however, a person perceives the work involved in making changes as outweighing the desired outcome, then motivation will decline. For example, if one has an item to return to a store that is far away from home or work (10-15 miles), one would need to decide whether the amount of money that he/she would get back is worth the amount of time and energy the process would involve. The more work ("pain") that is associated with the change

process, the less motivation the person will have.
This pain-pleasure principle controls our motivation.

For most people, the fear of loss/pain is much greater than the desire for pleasure/gain. One need only look at the plethora of advertisements geared toward pain prevention to confirm this insight. The typical cycle of dieting manifests the force of the pain/pleasure principle. The diet begins as a result of the pain associated with being overweight: a person looks in the mirror and thinks, "I can't stand how I look" or "I'm worried about my health." Then the person begins the diet by gaining education about different diets, cutting out certain foods, etc. As changes are made, the person begins to lose weight and as a result begins to feel better about his/her looks, to have more energy, and to feel healthier. The pleasure derived from this immediate success is very motivating, but soon the person notices that the weight loss is slowing down and begins to feel discouraged. In addition, the person encounters unrelated problems at work or in a relationship that add stress and pain. As the pleasure associated with the diet dwindles, and the diet proves to be powerless to affect the new sources of pain, the person loses motivation, binges, gains back a pound, decides the diet is too much work, and quits.

In your assessment with your client, it is helpful to determine whether he/she is more motivated by alleviating pain or pursuing pleasure. To help determine this, ask your client a question such as, "What does your work mean to you?" If the client replies, "It provides me with the money to have a great lifestyle," he/she is probably more motivated by seeking pleasure. If the client replies, "It keeps me from being poor and unable to pay my bills," he/she is probably more motivated by avoiding pain. This is an important determination, as you may be able to more effectively motivate your client when he/she seems to be at an impasse. At difficult times it may be more helpful to your client to say something like, "Let's make sure you don't go back to that place where you couldn't pay your bills," than, "Let's keep moving forward so your children can go to college."

How Quickly Can People Change?

People can change many aspects of themselves <u>instantly</u> and with relative ease, such as quitting drinking "cold turkey." According to psychologist James Prochaska, Professor of Psychology and Director of the Cancer Prevention Research Center at the University of Rhode Island in Kingston, "Twenty times as many people have quit smoking on their own, with no outside assistance, as those following a treatment program. Some psychological modalities also advertise their ability to help people make immediate changes in their lives. Eriksonian hypnosis and neurolinguistic programming (NLP) are two of the most common. More recent additions are EMDR, thought-field therapy, and emotional complex clearing. NLP, for example, can help clients eliminate a lifetime phobia in less than an hour -- something that in traditional therapies could take five years to work through. The only problem with these instantaneous changes is that many of them do not last. Although people can change in an instant, most people need long-term reinforcement or continuous maintenance to keep the changes in place. However, many of these techniques can be incorporated into longer-term programs. EMDR, for instance, has proven to be a remarkable method of inspiring sudden breakthroughs in insight. The change following these breakthroughs can still be a more gradual process. People are creatures of habit, and as a result, change is difficult. Coaches play a crucial role in providing the ongoing support and insight that accompany lasting change.

<u>Gradual Change</u>

Change is usually a gradual process that consists of many small steps. Often, people may be slowly working their way towards a goal without even realizing it. Prochaska found, "The average person makes the same New Year's resolution three years in a row before actually accomplishing it" (*American Health*). Prochaska works with people who wish to make life changes and has found that people rarely make sudden, dramatic shifts from one behavior to another. Instead, he has found that most people pass through a series of well-defined stages:

1.Pre-contemplation
2.Contemplation
3.Preparation
4.Action
5.Maintenance/Support
6.Termination/Relapse

In his book *Changing for Good* Prochaska explains that one may require several passes through these steps before succeeding. In fact, he compares the process of change as that of a "spiraling upward", or of climbing the Leaning Tower of Pisa: first, you walk up, but as you approach the lower part of each floor, you begin to head down, a few steps later you resume your ascent.

Many "Change Programs" have been unsuccessful because they failed to realize the importance of the preparation stages. It would be nice to start out your program with all your clients starting right away on their "action plan." In fact, when I began writing this book I thought Chapter 8 "Goal Setting" should show up much earlier. However, after a year or so of research I realized it had to be prefaced by seven other chapters!

Moreover, not everything can be changed. Most of our physical qualities cannot be changed, although they can be altered through artificial means, or, in some cases, manipulated by exercise, diet, or the intake of chemicals. An excellent study on this subject has been done by Martin Seligman, in his book *What You Can Change and What You Can't* (1994). Seligman discusses the term "human plasticity," or the ability to change. Those characteristics that are difficult (if not impossible) to change are called "heritable." Those that can be changed are called "changeable."

There has been much debate in the scientific community and in society as a whole about "nature vs. nurture." Perhaps the most effective work that has been done in attempting to determine which traits are heritable and which are changeable has been done with identical twins reared apart. What scientists have determined from these studies is that the most heritable traits (aside from physical characteristics) are IQ, mental speed, alcohol and drug abuse, natural weight, crime and conduct, job choice, and cheerfulness or depression. However, all of these can be altered to some extent. The recent studies show that IQ has an approximate heritability degree of .75. This means that 25% of our IQ comes from our actions and our experiences. The general consensus within the scientific and psychological communities now is that personality has approximately a .50 heritability degree. This opens the door for much opportunity for self-improvement, depending on the person's desire.

The change process can be approached according to any of the standard clinical models. My own approach is predominantly cognitive-behavioral, since I have found through both my studies and my experiences that this is often the most effective approach to motivation, and also the most practical approach in today's market which mandates short-term programs and encourages programs with tangible steps and measures. Nonetheless, I endeavor to incorporate elements from other models, especially psychoanalytic, since for many clients, change without insight tends to be meaningless and does not lead to long-term changes in outlook. I believe that the entire motivational process requires a combination of self-help and clinical theory, depending on each client's needs, in order to be most effective.

*If you're gonna make a change you have to operate
from a new belief
that says life happens not to me but for me.*
---Tony Robbins

Chapter Five:
Success Sabotage

All our dreams can come true if we have the courage to pursue them.
---Walt Disney

Psychological blocks to success range from common, mundane problems to severe blocks symptomatic of much larger conditions. Following are some of the most typical blocks encountered in a program. Following are the <u>seven major blockers</u> to one's movement toward their success, and ways to overcome each.

#1: It's Too Difficult

Even after a person has created a vision statement and action plan, one of the greatest roadblocks to success remains the lack of sustained, concerted effort. Most people are somewhat lazy: our natural tendency is to avoid stress and dedication, and, rather, to do what is fun, easy, and immediate. The most difficult thing to do is to discipline oneself to focus and concentrate, especially when a more immediately gratifying activity beckons. As an example, the American Dietary Association recently published the results of their 1997 nutrition survey, in which they reported that two-thirds of American adults do not eat a nutritious diet. The three main reasons people gave for not eating nutritiously were, 1) do not want to give up taste, 2) do not want to take the extra time, and 3) too difficult in general.

The coach should be understanding about the difficulty of the change process and validate the client's continued efforts. In this regard, coaches can prepare their clients for obstacles that they will inevitably encounter by warning them about the various types of sabotage that can occur. Coaches need to become aware of the times at which clients are getting off the path and confront the difficulty right away, since clients often lack awareness of their own straying. When clients stray, there is an opportunity for insight into the nature of the clients' blocks. Asking a client, "Did you notice anything this past week that got you off your path?" will assist the person in gaining insight into his/her own patterns of self-sabotage.

Usually what goes hand-in-hand with "it's too difficult," is "it's taking too long." This is probably the number one reason people do not stick with their goals. The payoff simply is not coming quickly enough. In fact, <u>most things of value in life take a long time to achieve</u>. Cognitive restructuring can be very beneficial during the struggle. Have clients look at their process as a long road, or journey. Ask them to describe the path they are on, and where it leads. Ask them where they are tempted to veer off, and where that path is likely to take them. Attempt to get clients to see the value of <u>staying true to their path</u>, if in fact, their desired success is somewhere along it, <u>even if it takes a long time</u>. Tony Robbins says, "You must have a long-term mindset. You need to be willing to endure some short-term pain or discomfort in order to achieve your goals." Remind clients that they don't have to <u>want</u> to do it, or <u>feel</u> like doing it, to do it! The saying "When the going gets tough, the tough get going," describes the inner strength one must "summons" in order to continue. It takes tremendous courage, determination and tenacity to continue, or get back up after a fall, during rough times. Encouragement and validation are especially important here.

#2: I Don't Deserve It

Self-esteem is an integral component of achieving one's goals. One can only pursue and keep what one thinks one deserves. Consequently, lack of self-esteem will sabotage success attempts. When one lacks self-esteem, an internalized critical inner voice will attempt to cancel one's ambitions through self-doubt and disbelief. In "Taming the Inner Critic" (*The California Coach*, Sept./Oct. 1997), Ernest Isaacs argues that if the Inner Critic is brought to one's attention, then this critical voice can be consciously distanced and refuted. Self-esteem work must be intertwined throughout the coaching process in order for the client to gain insight into why his or her success efforts have been thwarted in the past. With this insight, the client can arm him/herself with ammunition to stop the process of self-sabotage.

Life-style changes can greatly increase self-esteem. Such changes must be effected gradually and with great patience on the part of both client and coach. Basically, it is a process of becoming <u>aware</u> of and then <u>changing</u> unhealthy habits. The awareness is as critical as the subsequent change. The coach can give much-needed support during this process, as can friends and family members who are positive influences rather than saboteurs.

Another possible problem is the client's guilt about their own success or "havingness." Many clients describe a feeling of shame, or "awaiting punishment" when their lives are going well. Often, we hear things like, "Things are going <u>too</u> well. I'm just looking over my shoulder waiting for something bad to happen." It is as if every good thing must be followed by a bad thing. People talk about going through a "lucky streak" followed by a "streak of bad

38

luck." These kinds of statements need to be recognized as important, and dealt with therapeutically -- they may signal repressed guilt and shame that needs to be handled before one can move on.

Wayne Dyer, author of *The Sky's the Limit* does an excellent job of dealing with unhealthy guilt. He discusses the "guilt myth," wherein a person might believe "If I'm prospering, other people may be starving." The truth is, he explains, that the more you prosper, the better position you are in to help others in need. People will starve whether or not you prosper -- your "having more" does not take something away from someone else (unless of course, you've stolen it!). In fact, Dyer states, you can create better lives for others when you improve your own life.

#3: I Don't Have The Resources

Tony Robbins writes, "More than anything else, I believe it's our <u>decisions</u>, not the <u>conditions</u> of our lives, that determine our destiny." Many clients will give excuses as to why they cannot achieve their goals. Most of these excuses center around not having certain resources or advantages. It is true that some people have advantages, be they genetic, educational, environmental, monetary, or familial. But in *Simple Steps to Impossible Dreams*, Steven Scott insists that people who achieve "impossible dreams" are generally not very different in resources from the average person: "they <u>don't</u> have higher IQs; they have <u>not</u> been better educated; and they do not have better backgrounds than you. They simply learned and utilized some specific techniques that enabled them to 'dream big' and then to achieve those dreams." When your clients begin to talk about how others were blessed with advantages and they were not, you can remind them about the many people who, by making new decisions about their lives and pursuing their goals, overcame the odds and achieved extraordinary success that far exceeded their conditions.

#4: I Don't Have the Time

One of the most widespread problems is goal conflict--having multiple, conflicting goals, such as a teenager's desire for both total independence and a safe, nurturing home environment. Another example would be the adult who wants career success but wants to avoid any possibility for rejection. These conflicts tend to lead to inaction and depression, since the pursuit of one goal entails the betrayal of another goal. However, goal conflict does not imply a lack of motivation. Resolution of goal conflict stems from an awareness of the condition and subsequent discussion of the sources of the conflict. It is the coach's job to help the individual clarify values and prioritize goals: for example, the client can draw up a list of the pros and cons of possible paths and then come up with the best action to take at the current time.

Sometimes goals are not inherently contradictory, and in this case a less pressing goal can be achieved after a more immediately important one. If the goals are ongoing ones, such as being a top employee of a firm, spending time with one's children, and becoming an expert rock-climber, aspects of these various goals can be delegated: children can spend a little more time in daycare, so that the time one does spend with them is more freely given. Likewise, perhaps some of one's duties at work can be delegated; even if this means a slight cut in pay, it might be worth it if it allows one to continue a job while simultaneously being a good parent and pursuing an interest in rock climbing.

Coaches should be aware that goal conflict can arise legitimately, but it can also serve as an excuse for abandoning goals before they are complete. A focus for coaching in this case might be time management, values clarification, and prioritizing. Assisting the client in creating a "Life Time Line" can be very helpful, so they can see that they have time left to achieve many more of their goals.

#5: I Can't Do It

A widespread theory to explain the prevalence of internal blocks is Seligman's theory of learned helplessness: the theory that individuals develop feelings of helplessness when they feel that the consequences of their behavior occur independently of their action and are thus beyond their control. This leads such individuals to lose motivation and to extend the feeling of helplessness beyond this particular situation so that it becomes a general condition. Testing has proven that the theory is only true when the cause is viewed by the individual as internal, stable and global -- an inherent deficit. More common than a general sense of learned helplessness is the sense of helplessness in particular areas. The role of the coach is to assist clients in reassessing their strengths and learning new self-statements regarding personal strength and confidence. Interventions include reviewing the client's past successes, and creating positive affirmations and self-statements. For more on this subject, see the section "I'm Afraid."

#6: They Don't Want Me To

A hypersensitivity to the role of others in one's pursuit of a goal tends to impede motivation by giving one the sense that these others control one's situation and that as a result one's effort is contingent upon their participation, encouragement, and acceptance. Moreover, it can be tempting to blame others for one's own lack of motivation, claiming that they will be jealous, angry, or overly needy if one succeeds. Doing so may seem to be a means of absolving oneself of culpability for one's failures, but it has the more dangerous aspect of depriving one of autonomy: if it is others who are to blame for one's failures, then it is these same others who control one's successes. It is important for the coach to get at the heart of the client's fears. When a person is blocked because of fear of what others will think, focusing on the goal of "developing my true self" becomes a compelling replacement for the fear of "others' disapproval." Failure of the coach and client to handle <u>this one issue</u> - sabotage by others -- can <u>sabotage the entire motivational or helping process</u>!

The best way to resist sabotage by others is to develop a sense of autonomy. Coaches can help clients assess who is helping them become independent and confident, and who is hindering the process. Coaches can help clients organize their lives so as to <u>minimize the power and influence of people who are likely to sabotage their chances for success and look instead toward those who are supportive</u>. Undertaking a task in the context of a supportive, nurturing environment increases motivation, both because these conditions foster a sense of one's own ability and because one internalizes the desire to please supporters by performing well.

A well known business consultant says, "Run, don't walk, I repeat RUN, DON'T WALK, from negative people!" But what if one <u>cannot</u> leave (or it is not in their overall best interest to leave) the people who are their greatest source of discouragement? In these cases, the coach can assist clients in learning how to elicit support. Prochaska discusses the idea of "enlisting " or "eliciting" helping relationships

throughout his book. He believes that most people
<u>do not know how</u> to help, and yet helping
relationships are of <u>primary value</u> to self changers. It
is often up to the client to teach their family, friends,
co-workers, roommates, etc how they can be the most
helpful.

On the other hand, some clients have
"supporters" who exude tremendous pressure on
them to achieve a particular goal, which may or may
not be the client's goal. For example, the well-
meaning mother who tells her daughter, "You know
you really should go into interior design . . . you're
very artistic . . . you have a gift . . . you shouldn't let
it go to waste…" and so on. <u>Pressure creates
resistance</u>. The more one is pressured to do
something, the more difficult it seems to become.
The classic example is the "chronic underachieving
child" from the "high achieving parents." Clients of
all ages need to learn how to set limits with people
who pressure, and again, teach them how to be
supportive.

The power of a support system cannot be
emphasized enough. One only has to watch the
"Academy Awards" and the celebrities who have
climbed to the top of their profession (no easy feat!),
and listen to their acceptance speeches. They almost
never mention the difficulties, the processes, how
they overcame their own sabotages and adversities --
rather they spend their few moments thanking the
people who supported them -- and they all have them.
I have devoted an entire chapter (Chapter 9) to the
social aspects of motivation.

<u>#7: I'm Afraid</u>

Most people fear the unknown. Fear keeps
people persisting in unhappy and dysfunctional
situations, because they know that changing the
situation will lead to the unknown, which may be

even more painful than what they are currently experiencing. Their fear may be founded or unfounded, but it needs to be examined in the context of reality testing to determine now great the risk really is. Coaches have the crucial role of assisting clients in determining whether the changes that they are considering are likely to increase their likelihood of leading more satisfying, happier lives. Will the woman who is now being emotionally abused by her husband be better off with a divorce? How will she cope? Can she support herself and her children financially? How will the move affect her children? Where will they live? Is the separation worth the risk, or is there a better way? It is the coach's job to explore these alternatives with the client.

Most fears that inhibit motivation stem from low self-esteem. In this regard, the fear of failure and the fear of success are integrally connected. Atkinson's "Michigan Studies of Fear and Failure" states that the tendency to avoid failure seems to dampen the effort to perform well. Consequently, fearing failure is counter-productive, since it essentially furthers the likelihood of failure. For some, the fear of failure is so great that it seems safer not to attempt anything at all. Often such people have experienced a failure that felt devastating and that they haven't worked through. Attempting something new is thus viewed as taking the risk of repeating such a crushing disappointment.

The coach can be instrumental in helping clients assess past fears and failures and work through them. A cognitive restructuring technique is to substitute the phrase "learning experience" for "failure." However, the technique is only useful within a limited context, since abolishing the word "failure" altogether similarly renders meaningless the concept of success. Perhaps a more useful rephrasing is Steven Scott's, who defines failure as "an _event_ in which you did not achieve your desired outcome."

The danger of believing in failure is that people tend to generalize: "I failed, therefore I'm a failure." Thus Scott's emphasizing of "event" is a means of putting the failure into perspective, as a single event, rather than a life prognosis. Likewise, the purpose of using the phrase "learning experience" is to help the client realize that what seems like a failure is not an end to everything but part of a larger <u>growth process</u>. The concept can be similarly applied to success, since ideally successes are not ending points but milestones en route to other successes. In a competitive society such as the U.S., we can be brainwashed into thinking that everything is either a win or a loss. Right or wrong. One up or one down. Good or bad. Because much of mental health has to do with our "perception" of what happens to us, we need to assist our clients in refraining from this type of splitting and help them transfer to more positive thoughts.

Coaches can further assist clients by encouraging them to do research on new goals at which they fear they will fail. Through research, clients can, to some extent determine the likelihood of success and assess whether their fears are founded. For instance, if the client is afraid of applying to a particular graduate school, the client can look at statistics on what percentage of applicants are accepted into the program, what percentage of those accepted complete the program, and what percentage of those that complete the program successfully find jobs.

Like the fear of failure, the fear of criticism and the fear of change lead to inaction, since that is the safer route when low self-esteem leads one to believe that criticism is inevitable and change can only bring disaster. The fear of criticism further reflects low self-esteem in that it reflects an over-dependence on the opinion of an outsider, a lack of self-respect and confidence in one's own abilities.

Fear of success occurs when a person has such self-doubt that success brings with it overwhelming anxiety -- a sense that the success is not deserved, that it cannot last, and that disaster is imminent. Often in such cases, people will purposefully destroy the success so as to end the anxiety that accompanies it, feeling that known failure is better than the prolonged anticipation of failure. We know too well the scenario of those who rose to the top so rapidly, and so unprepared, that they self medicated their anxiety with drugs and/or alcohol (often to their own demise).

The fears of failure and success are blocks that, with patience and time, can be confronted and overcome (unless they are part of a larger, more severe personality disorder, in which case they should be treated by an expert in that particular area). If the problem relates to a specific goal, begin by helping your client to choose tasks related to this goal that are neither too large nor too challenging (although there must be some challenge for success to be accompanied by a sense of accomplishment). Once success has been proven with respect to small, simple tasks, the individual's confidence increases and the fear of failure diminishes because success has been proven. Take for example the reclusive, awkwardly shy teenage boy who gets his first job and suddenly begins to express himself more freely. The act of undertaking the pursuit of a goal can in itself build self-esteem, whether or not the goal itself is eventually achieved. As individuals become increasingly confident about their abilities, they become ready to take on larger challenges.

Psychological studies have shown that people may regret actions more than inactions at first, but over a longer period of time they come to regret inactions more than actions. Gilovich found that when elderly people were asked about their greatest lifetime regrets, 63 percent of the regrets were about inaction. Often, communicating this statistic to clients can help them overcome fears and doubts about action and feel readier to take risks and pursue goals.

If you drink much from a bottle marked 'poison,' it is almost certain to disagree with you, sooner or later.
---Lewis Carroll from *Alice and Wonderland*

Chapter Six: Thought and Attitude Transformation

Nothing in the world can take the place of persistence.
Talent will not; nothing is more common than unsuccessful men with talent. Genius will not; unrewarded genius is almost a proverb. Education will not; the world is full of educated derelicts. Persistence and determination alone are omnipotent.
---Calvin Coolidge

Influences on Change

There are many factors that play a part in one's ability to change. Martin Seligman, in his studies on human plasticity, as reported in his book, *What You Can Change and What You Can't*, found the following to be the primary influences that affect the ability to change:

--Immediate situation (how effectively one reacts to the situation)
--Removed situations (life history, childhood, race, cultural system, etc.)
--Genetics
--Self discipline (willpower, ambition, initiative, determination, persistence, etc.)
--Character
--Personal belief in one's ability to change

The more advantages one has in these areas, the easier it will be. The challenge for the coach is to work like a detective to uncover which one of these influences has had the most impact on the person's inability to change in the past and work on this area. According to Carl Rogers, the crucial element that enables client change is the empathic attitude of the coach. While it is important to realize how much power the coach does have to encourage and facilitate change, it is also important to focus on the client's particular background. Each individual possesses personal traits that will enable or disable him/her to develop motivation and remain motivated even after the course of a program has ended.

Developing Ambition

Ambition is a critical component of achievement. In order to pursue one's life goals, one must first become ambitious. This means breaking out of the comfortable familiarity of routine termed the "comfort zone" by the authors of *Do It! Let's Get Off Our Buts*. But how does one get ambition? Steven Scott describes the process in terms of an "awakening": realizing that we have been "programmed for mediocrity" and then realizing that this prior programming does not doom us to continuing to abide by this mediocrity. As Sarah Breathnach argues in her book, *Simple Abundance*, perhaps ambition is already within us:

Ambition is achievement's soul mate. Action is the matchmaker that brings these affinities together so that sparks can begin to fly and we can set the world on fire.... Just as electricity can be life enhancing or destructive, so can ambition. What ambition really needs is a new press agent. The only time we ever hear about her is when she's blamed for somebody's downfall.... But what if we are supposed to be ambitious? What if our refusal to channel our ambitions for our highest good, the highest good of those we love and the rest of the world, is the real corruption of Power? Think of all that could be accomplished if women cherished their ambitions and brought them into the Light where they belong. Think of how our lives could be transformed if we

*respected ambition and gave grateful thanks for
being entrusted with such a miraculous gift.*

According to Breathnach's theory, the coach can assume the client has suppressed ambition. The challenge in the coaching process, then, is to bring to light the ambition that is within the client. This ambition may be difficult to find, as it may have been squelched for many years. Often, however, all it takes is to give the client permission to bring it up. In order to counter the common tendency to think of ambition, or drive, as a negative characteristic, the coach can validate ambition as a positive attribute--a gift--when used for good, in the pursuit of one's goals. When the client's ideas about ambition have been transformed into a positive framework, a motivational breakthrough often follows.

Developing healthy ambition is often about finding a balance. Optimistic thinking has proven to be a major factor in self-motivation. Nonetheless, we all know of clients who are over-optimistic and over-ambitious. These people are often called "dreamers" or "serial enthusiasts." They move from place to place, job to job, relationship to relationship, hobby to hobby, each time announcing that "THIS IS THE ONE!" Ambitious people often have over-ambitious goals as well as over-ambitious time lines. They only feel good if they achieve large goals, so they lose sight of the smaller goals. They are too impatient to work on the smaller sub-goals and the often tedious steps involved in getting to the larger goals. This is why they are constantly changing. As soon as it starts to get difficult or frustrating, or if it seems to take too long or is too much work, they move on to the next "great idea." When a client says he/she has stopped progress on a certain goal because "I've changed my mind" the coach needs to assess if the client is <u>really</u> saying, "It got too hard," or "It's taking too long."

On the other hand, pessimists worry about doing things perfectly and never seem able to make a move. They continually use their imagination to visualize worst case scenarios, then conclude that those scenarios are so hopeless that there is no cause for action. As coaches, we need to be able to assess these patterns and intervene.

On a continuum between overly optimistic and overly pessimistic, there is a healthy medium. Healthy people who find themselves thinking too optimistically or pessimistically will challenge their own thoughts. They will look at both sides of the coin and debate them until they feel they have a realistic idea of how to proceed. If this course of action does not achieve the desired results, they will alter or modify it until it does. It is important to help your clients become realists, to get to a point between over-optimism and pessimism where they can debate the pros and cons of various actions and assess likely outcomes.

Moreover, ambition does not just spring up automatically. Often, one must begin a task because of self-discipline rather than intrinsic motivation. But if one can develop the discipline to begin, motivation will often follow. Extrinsic motivation can be internalized, or interjected, and with the passage of time, as one adjusts to new tasks and becomes pleased with the results of new successes, intrinsic motivation can develop.

Controlled Focus

Tony Robbins, one of the greatest contributors to motivational thought transformation in the self-help movement, writes, "In order to succeed, you must have a long-term focus." He believes that in order to gain any valuable, long-term pleasure, one must break through some short-term pain. This begins with the decision to overcome the discomfort of short-term pain. Robbins speaks of the principle of "concentration of power" or "controlled focus." He believes that people can achieve more than they realize when then focus their intentions on their goals. His delineation of the thought transformation process involves three steps:

1) Raise Your Standards: Decide what you will accept and what you will not accept for your life.
2) Change Your Limiting Beliefs: Develop a sense of confidence that you can and will meet your new standards.
3) Change Your Strategy: The best strategy is to find a role model, someone who is already getting the results you want, and tap into their knowledge.

"Your life changes," says Robbins, "the moment you make a <u>new</u>, <u>congruent</u>, and <u>committed</u> decision." Brian Tracy reiterates Robbins' point about long-term focus in his book, *Secrets of Success,* and goes on to emphasize the feelings of confidence, mastery, and self-esteem that ensue when one achieves sustained concentration.

Cognitive Strategies for Self-Defeating Statements

Positive affirmations can replace former negative ones, if a person hears them repeatedly. The coach is in a position to give new messages over and over, since usually there is weekly contact with the client. When providing motivational support, the coach needs to avoid making statements like "That's because your father told you that you would never succeed at anything" too often. The coach needs to make more positive than negative statements in the session. A statement such as the one just mentioned should always be followed with a question such as, "How are you succeeding at something today?" Wayne Dyer, the popular self-help author, promotes the idea of "The Sky's the Limit" by showing how working through self-defeating labels and behaviors, people can build confidence and self-esteem so that there are no limits to what they can achieve. Require the clients to come up with their own positive statements about themselves. When a client makes a negative statement about him/her self, ask him/her (gently) to immediately replace it with a positive one. Another cognitive technique is known as "Stop Think." Tell the client that as soon as a negative thought comes into his/her head, immediately think "STOP!" and change over to a positive thought that has been prepared to replace the negative one.

Useful words to incorporate in thought transformation are: focus, concentration, self-discipline, willpower, dedication, persistence, perseverance, commitment, determination, courage, dedication.

Some of these attributes come naturally and some take more work. The coach can instill these concepts by using the words frequently to validate progress: tell a client who has just accomplished something, "Wow, that shows perseverance." More information on affirmations can be found in Chapter 10, "Spiritual Aspects of Motivation."

Deriving Inspiration from Stories of Others who Overcame Adversity

Hearing the personal histories of people who overcame hardship and proved wrong those who had given up on them can be an inspiring experience for many. Relating these stories to clients in a program is an excellent way to assist them in working through their blocks as well as inspiring them. The reason this strategy works so well is that people learn from imitation. It is helpful to have a model of a person (or several people) with whom one can identify: someone who has had similar struggles and has overcome them. One is thus led to think, if so-and-so could do it, why can't I? The stories have the effect of making one identify with a community of survivors, of confident people who believed in themselves and achieved success because of their determination. Following are some sample stories:

*Motivational author and speaker Tony Robbins contends that his own rags-to-riches story proves that success "requires internal commitment, not external credentials." Robbins, who earns up to $60,000 a day conducting corporate seminars and $12 million a year selling motivational books and tapes, is a high school graduate with no formal training, no professional license, and no academic degree. For Robbins, confidence and determination are the crucial elements that enable success.

*Albert Einstein was born with a misshapen head and an abnormally large body. He learned to talk so late that his parents feared he was mentally retarded. He was also so withdrawn that one governess named him "Father Bore." Because he found schoolwork (especially memorization) tedious, he paid little attention. As a result, many of his teachers dismissed him as dimwitted. He dropped out of high school and failed a technical college entrance exam. When his interest was piqued, however, he proved to be a genius. His calling just happened to be higher mathematics (*Biography Magazine*). No one is successful at everything. A critical component of motivation and success is finding one's niche, one's passion.

*Thomas Muster, an Austrian professional tennis player, was ranked sixth in the world. He had just won the semi-finals of the Lipton International Tennis Tournament and was scheduled to play in the men's finals the next day. That night, while putting his tennis bag in the trunk of his car, a drunk driver hit him and shattered his knee so badly that after his surgery, the doctors told him he might never walk again. He did come back, however, and was able to rise back up to his sixth place ranking in the world. Muster's story demonstrates the importance of being adaptive as well as determined. Muster's life was clearly changed by his accident, but rather than succumbing to this setback, he adapted to the new circumstances with even greater determination (*Biography Magazine*).

*Michael Jordan, one of the best basketball players of all time, continues to amaze us by breaking his own personal records over and over. He has said that what motivates him is the challenge. When he hears a sportscaster (or a competitor) express doubts that Jordan can rise to the occasion or state that his team is not favored to win, he simply hears it as a challenge, which serves to increase his motivation to prove himself capable and to prove his challengers wrong. Many clients will come in having encountered similar criticism from others: someone in their past told them they couldn't do it, someone told them they were a failure, they had negative labels placed on them by significant adults during their childhood. Jordan's determination exemplifies the way in which these negative statements can be used as a positive motivational force, if they are viewed as a challenge rather than as confirmation of unavoidable failure.

Using Life Traumas or Difficulties as Motivators

As the anecdote about Muster exemplifies, life traumas have the potential to work as motivators rather than inhibitors. One almost always encounters obstacles in the pursuit of one's goals. Overcoming obstacles -- particularly large ones -- proves one's determination and makes one's attainment of the final goal that much more meaningful. In *Imperfect Control*, Judith Viorst writes,

*Studies of victimization have found that most
of us, until we have been victimized, share three
basic, often unconscious, assumptions:*

*We assume that we are personally
invulnerable.*
*We assume that the world we live in is
comprehensible.*
*We assume that we are essentially
worthwhile.*

Victimization deprives us of this sense of certainty. As the title of Viorst's book suggests, no one is always in control of life. The assumptions that Viorst lists as characterizing people who have never been victimized suggest an attitude of taking life for granted. Although it is certainly not to be wished for, the experience of trauma can thus lead to increased motivation, because it robs one of these assumptions, forcing one to reevaluate what in life is important and what is worth pursuing.

The notion of hardship as leading to increased motivation is affirmed in Gail Sheehy's *Pathfinders*. She writes, "Repeated to a striking degree in the histories of the most satisfied adults was a history of a troubled period during late childhood or adolescence, when many rated themselves as very unhappy. Anyone who overcomes a difficult childhood is likely to acquire that key characteristic-- a concentration of optimism--and quite possibly an orientation toward the present and future rather than an emphasis on the past."

It is not what happens to us that influences our motivation so much as our <u>perceptions</u> of what happens and the manner in which we choose to act in response. In terms of thought transformation, perpetual victims see life in terms of "Why me?" and "I can't, because..." whereas recovering victims see

life in terms of "What can I do with this?"
Unhappiness and discomfort can be calls to action.

At times, we all become overwhelmed. An effective coach, however, has to be able to help people see the end goal, to take one step at a time, rather than being overwhelmed by the issues.
---Byron and Catherine Pulsifer, from *Common Traits of a Coach*

<u>Chapter Seven:</u>
<u>Personal Vision or Mission</u>

A dream is a wish your heart makes.
---Cinderella

A personal vision is what motivates a person to set goals. Therefore, it is important to create a vision before attempting to set goals or create an action plan. Motivational experts call personal vision many different things, such as primary aim, main purpose, life mission, and core intention. The reason I prefer the term personal vision is that it implies a picture, and it is very helpful to create a picture of how one's life will look when one's mission is accomplished. Perhaps the client will not have an end goal, but rather a process or life journey, and this is fine. Either way, it is important for the client to write out a statement and either draw or describe a picture of his/her vision.

One coach's vision statement is "to assist people in living happier, more productive lives in ways that will benefit the whole of society." She describes it in visual terms this way:

I see my clients working through their processes in treatment with me, coming back each session having had breakthroughs, changing and growing toward better mental, emotional, physical, and spiritual health. I see them getting happier and more positive about their ability to control their lives, getting smarter about how to conduct their lives in healthier ways. I see them becoming more caring and loving toward others, while setting healthy limits for themselves. I see them becoming more productive and positive role models in society. I see them helping make the world a better place. I see all people from all nations working together to help each other achieve their goals. I see peace, safety, good health, and good will.

This is an example of a career-related vision. Many people only have a career mission and have never thought about having a mission in other areas of their lives. Of course, it is fine to have one main vision statement for one's life, but because people are complex and we encourage balance, it is healthy to have a separate mission statement for each of the main areas of life. I recommend creating a vision statement for each of the 6 areas we have listed in the next chapter: physical/emotional health; relationship/marriage; family; professional/career; social/political; spiritual; leisure/recreation.

The 3 V's: Values, Vision and Voice

I use the term "the three V's"- values, vision, voice. First, people must determine what their core values are when determining their goals. Second, they need to give their goals a vision, and third, they need to give their goals a voice. The difference between goals and a vision is that goals are activities you want to accomplish and a vision is what motivates you to set those goals. Thus before goal-setting work can be done, it is important to define the client's vision and then to formulate it in terms of a mission. The client determines his/her mission according to several criteria: the mission will have something to do with the client's value system, past experiences (either very negative or very positive), skills, talents, abilities, interests, and sources of joy. Finally, the mission reflects the client's self-concept and perceptions about his/her ability to accomplish goals.

The "PPPP" Principle

A follow-up to the three V's is what I call the "PPPP Principle." The P's stand for Prophecy, Passion, Power and Propulsion. Once clients have defined a personal vision -- a <u>prophecy</u> of what they wish for and will achieve -- simply focusing on this vision will provide them with feeling of <u>passion</u>. Their feeling of passion will give them the <u>power</u> to <u>propel</u> them into action.

It's only when we give to ourselves as passionately as
we give of ourselves
that we create the life we want and deserve.
---Suze Orman

Chapter Eight:
Setting Goals & Creating an Action Plan

It is a paradoxical but profoundly true and important principle of life that the most likely way to reach a goal is to be aiming not at that goal itself but at some more ambitious goal beyond it.
---Arnold Toynbee

Setting Goals

Goals are born from vision. Denis Waitley, author of *The New Dynamics of Goal Setting*, believes so strongly that people cannot succeed without goals that he makes the bold statement, "All successful people set goals." Developing goals is predominantly a matter of structure and organization. A poster on the wall of a gym states, "A goal is a dream with a deadline." Coaches can help clients feel motivated to set goals by encouraging them to construct meaning around the goal, asking the clients, "How will the attainment of this goal change your life, make your life better?" Conversely, coaches can act as a "reality measure" by assisting clients in setting appropriate, attainable goals and facilitating the communication of these goals to others. If the client has a tendency toward grandiosity, the coach can be the reality check and assist in toning down the terms of explanation. If the client has a tendency to be shy and humble, the coach can assist in assertiveness.

Richard Suinn, Ph.D., past President of the American Psychological Association is a sports psychologist -- the first to serve on a U.S. Olympic sports medicine team. He states, "Instead of just getting athletes 'psyched up,' we prefer to help them become more definite about why they're doing what

they're doing now, even though their eventual goal --
say winning a gold medal -- may be a few years
down the road. Goal setting helps to bring the future
a little closer by breaking it down into steps to take
this week, next week, and next month. That way
athletes can chart their progress, keeping in mind
where they're eventually going to end up. It enables
those who are feeling that they want to give up to
stay with the program."

Creating an Action Plan

Let's now assume that your client has set
some healthy goals. For a goal to be carried out, an
action plan must be developed, thereby breaking
down the goal into specific subgoals, which divide a
goal into more manageable steps. The plan can be
compared to a battle plan, wherein winning the war is
the long-range goal and the battles are the shorter
units that must be completed successfully to ensure
the final victory. The coach can also use metaphors
such as training for a marathon or climbing a
mountain.

In *Simple Steps to Impossible Dreams*, Steven
Scott refers to this process as the "Dream Conversion
Process," and divides it into the following steps:

1) Define your dream in writing.
2) Convert your dream into specific goals.
3) Convert each goal into specific steps.
4) Convert each step into specific tasks.
5) Assign a projected time or date to complete each
task.

Prioritizing

Often, people are unable to begin pursuing a
goal because they have too many goals, not all of
which can be undertaken at once. For more on the

subject of conflicting goals, see the section "I Don't Have the Time" in Chapter 5. If goals are prioritized, the more important ones can be tackled first. Undertaking these goals one at a time overcomes the daunting specter that the mass of them together presented. Less critical or immediate goals can be pursued later. Writing out a time line is one way of remembering and committing to later goals while still pursuing only a limited number at the present time.

Keeping a journal of steps and sub-goals that have been met is a tangible way to measure progress and feel good about it.

Setting Sub-goals, and Tasks

Sub-goals strengthen motivation because they make an activity manageable and accessible. When a larger goal is divided into sub-goals, it becomes a series of incremental tasks rather than one overwhelming project. The idea has been expressed in many slogans that may appeal to your clients and that they can repeat to themselves to increase and sustain their motivation to subdivide and stick with their goals:

By the inch it's a cinch, by the yard it's hard.
One day at a time (From Alcoholics Anonymous).
Just put one foot in front of the other.
Nothin' to it but to do it!

Sometimes, it is more profitable to block out the daunting, long-range picture of one's goals in order to focus more completely on the immediate steps that need to be undertaken.

Maintenance

Maintenance includes measuring sub-goals, assessing habits and distributing rewards. This is an extremely important part of goal attainment. The coach needs to assist clients in measuring their progress, encourage them to stay on their path, and validate (or encourage a reward system) for their progress (Prochaska). When sub-goals and tasks are completed, they can be crossed off the plan. When they are completed on time, they can have a happy face drawn next to them. It is important for a person's motivation to measure the amount of work accomplished and mark its place on the plan, as this demonstrates that there is progress being made. Success breeds success. When a person feels that he/she has mastered a project, he/she will be more motivated to start the next one. The coach has an important role in helping to measure progress, validating the progress, and encouraging the client to continue doing that which is working.

Furthermore, the coach can help guide the client's progress. When the individual begins to veer off course, the coach can gently nudge them back to the path. An excellent way to do this is to remind clients that staying on the path will give them what they say they really want. Each task that is completed needs to be praised, and each time the client gets back on track, this needs to be validated. The coach should keep reminding the client of the benefits of staying with the plan. Task completion creates feelings of self-esteem. Goal achievement leads to feelings of self-confidence.

Prochaska's research has shown that subjects utilizing a "reward" system have better results. The coach and client together can come up with ideas for rewards. Something as small as "positive self statements" as self reward, can often be sufficient. Have the client come up with their own ideas to incorporate healthy rewards for themselves as each sub-goal is accomplished.

<u>Termination and/or Relapse</u>

When to terminate the program is a difficult question. It depends mostly on the client's initial goals for him or herself as well as the perception of his/her success. The decision to remain in a program is ultimately up to the client to decide. We provide some guidelines around what is the usual, customary and reasonable time to begin termination in Chapter 11. Termination is usually discussed often, throughout the process, so that it does not come as a surprise to either the client or the coach when it happens.

Since the goal attainment process is rarely a smooth, linear progression, we cannot expect clients who are on track during termination, to remain on track forever. Coaches need to sufficiently educate clients about relapse and reverting back to "old habits" so that they will be prepared if it happens. Also discussed in Chapter 11, is the concept of "intermittent coaching," so that when or if the client regresses or relapses, he/she knows he/she is welcome to return to coaching to get back on track.

If you can't figure out your purpose, figure out your passion.
For your passion will lead you right into your purpose.
---Bishop T.D. Jakes

My father gave me the greatest gift anyone could give another person, he believed in me.
---Jim Valvano, Basketball Coach

Social Motivation

The presence of others as a factor that increases a person's desire to perform well is a phenomenon known as social motivation. The movie *Alive* is based on the amazing, true story of a South American rugby team whose plane crashed in the Andes en route to a tournament in Santiago. Those few who survived said their courage came from not only their fear of death but also their will to see their families again. Emphasizing the social component of motivation, they all stated that it was the constant encouragement of their teammates that forced them to stay alive. Likewise, Albert Einstein mused, "Strange is our situation here on earth--we are here for a short visit--why? I don't know. I sense a divine calling that I am here for the sake of other humans and unknown soldiers whose fate is connected by a bond of sympathy." For Adler, the social context was so critical that he contended that people could not be studied in isolation, since the choices that people make are always formulated within a social context.

The social context in which goals are pursued has a direct effect on motivation. The presence of others can increase a person's desire to perform well, a phenomenon referred to as social facilitation. An example would be an employee who is being watched by a boss and co-employees while performing a task. Conversely, working on a project in a group can lead to a decrease in individual motivation, since the pressure rests on the group as a whole rather than on the individual. This phenomenon is known as social loafing.

It is important to be careful of negative social influences. Sometimes, one has family members or friends who are less successful and as a result try to hold one back. For many individuals, the pursuit of new goals leads to resistance from certain people close to them. This is because their new motivation and energy makes other people uncomfortable, either because it reminds them that they have given up on their own dreams, or because they are envious, or because they fear losing their "known/familiar" relationship with their friend, or because they think they are being more "realistic" when they express criticism and doubt. It is possible that these people's doubts are legitimate and that the individual's goals are problematic or unrealistic. In this case, the coach is in a unique position to assess the situation and assist the client in determining the intent and appropriateness of criticism from the client's social network.

Role Models

Role models can be an integral part of developing confidence with respect to new goals. For instance, a Latina student who will be the first person in her family to go to college will have a greater sense of confidence about her ability to succeed if she is introduced to a supportive Latina who comes from a similar background, has successfully completed college, and has embarked on a rewarding career based on her academic success in college.

Role models can be found through research as well as personal contact. If your client is in need of examples of people who have succeeded at goals similar to his/hers, you can encourage the client to go to a library or bookstore and do research. If the client doesn't know of any particular people to research, he/she can begin by reading biographies.

Mentors, Sponsors, Teachers, and Coaches

Mentors play a critical role in helping people overcome hardship and adversity. Alcoholics Anonymous uses a sponsor system in which new members are matched with sponsors who have had similar experiences and who have overcome similar problems. In *Pathfinders* (1981), her detailed study of people who succeed in life and remain optimistic and motivated even in the face of adversity, Gail Sheehy writes, "Even when pathfinders had an absent or severely flawed parent--and many of them did--somewhere they found a person who became a transformative figure for them...Instead of allowing a less than ideal set of parents to set them back permanently, the potential pathfinders usually gravitated toward another figure who did have purpose and direction and who offered something healing, cohering, possibly even inspiring."

Successful people discover a way of drawing from the environment what they need, finding supporters who can help them overcome obstacles and can serve as mentors. Moreover, such supporters provide a sense of structure in a person's life, thereby enabling them to take risks and make important changes. A coach can help clients figure out who in their lives are these supporters. The coach can serve <u>temporarily</u> as a mentor, sponsor, teacher and coach, however, it is important for <u>long lasting success</u> that clients find others to serve this role as well. Forming a supportive social network reinforces the ideas discussed in a program and helps keep the client moving forward in the pursuit of goals.

<u>**Partners**</u>

Partnering and teamwork, rather than leading to social loafing, can also lead to greater motivation if one feels truly committed to the other team members. Even with a low sense of self-esteem, one can go beyond these self-doubts because of the desire to succeed not only for oneself but for the other members of the team. Having a partner can increase the motivation of both people, because they can profit from each other's energy and motivation and because the partnership forms a larger unit than the self to which each partner becomes committed and for which each feels responsible. The only caveat is that each of the partners should maintain a level of independence. In a co-dependent partnership, one of the partners needs to be needed and thus focuses predominantly on the needs of the other person rather than the self or the partnership. In a dependent relationship, one of the partners needs help and relies on the other to provide it. Unlike mentoring or coaching, partnering should be a balanced relationship. If a client is part of a co-dependent or dependent partnership, the coach can help establish as a goal for this client the aim of becoming more independent.

In the corporate setting, more emphasis is being placed on "teamwork" and creation of "working teams." This concept has been shown to be much more productive than when workers previously worked in isolation in their cubicles. Team members can provide additional motivation and support, however, they can also impede progress if they have a negative attitude. Team members can become more united and less irritated with each other if they keep their <u>focus on the goal</u>.

Some people need more social support than others do: some individuals work better alone, others work better as part of a team. If the client is someone who works better as part of a team, goals should be tailored toward preference. One of the main functions of the coach is to provide the support of weekly contact. However, it is important that the coach limit his or her own role as a social support so that the client does not become dependent.

Fly in "V" Formation

Research shows that we are shaped largely by our interactions with others. Whether we have a long conversation with a friend or simply place an order at a restaurant, every interaction makes a difference. The results of our encounters are rarely neutral; they are almost always positive or negative. Remember, motivation is based mostly on "VEE" – Values, Enjoyment and Empowerment. When I think of "VEE" I think of a flock of geese flying into their traditional "V" formation. Engineers have learned that each bird, by flapping its wings, creates an uplift for the bird that follows. Together the whole flock gains about 70 percent greater flying range than if they were journeying alone.

In pursuing your goals, especially difficult ones, you cannot afford the luxury of a negative thought! You must devote a huge amount of your energy to motivating yourself and pursuing your goal. You don't have enough energy to ward off negative energy and still pursue your goal with fervor.

If you feel someone is not giving you the support you would like in pursuit of your new goals, you should first assess whether their doubts are valid. Is it possible that these doubts are legitimate and that your goals are either too rushed, problematic or unrealistic? If this is not the case, and you feel that they are not being supportive due to other reasons, you should discuss this with them, but you should not allow their discomfort to stand in the way of you achieving your goals.

This being said, you need to know that the people who are close to you usually do want to support you but don't know how. You need to teach them how. You may need to give them the exact step-by-step process to use. Above all, I ask the people closest to me to be supportive, validating and encouraging. If they slip into negativity, I simply imagine I have a mirror in front of me and their words bounce off me and reflect back onto them. I state, "I only hear positives."

It is imperative for your success that you surround yourself with positive thinkers. It is difficult enough to be a positive thinker, so without encouragement and validation from others your progress will be impeded. Ask others in your life to "catch" you when you slip into negative thinking and self-doubt. Ask them to force you to restate your words into a more positive statement. Ask them to remind you of how far you've come and how much you have already accomplished.

Once you've done the mental work, there comes a point you have to throw yourself into the action and put your heart on the line. That means not only being brave, but being passionate towards yourself, your teammates and your opponents.
---Phil Jackson

Chapter Ten:
Spiritual Aspects of Motivation

Our lives are what our thoughts create.
---Wayne Dyer

Spirituality, as I use the term, includes not just overt religious belief but encompasses more general aspects of belief, hope, and faith. Abraham Twerski defines it in the following terms:

There are many features over and above pure intellect that characterize us and distinguish us from other forms of life. We have the capacity to learn from the past, contemplate the purpose of our existence, bring about self-improvement, think about the consequences of our actions, delay gratification, and make moral choices. All these uniquely human characteristics comprise the <u>spirit</u>*.... When we exercise these capacities we are being spiritual.*

Thus, spirituality addresses the moral and ethical component of existence, and, in terms of motivation, encompasses the question of <u>*life purpose and improvement*</u>.

There is a current conflict between two schools of thought, both equally popular today in self-help literature. The first advocates self-determination -- the ability of the individual to change his/her life in whatever ways desired and the second advocates belief in a higher power -- the acceptance of the role of fate or divine influence in determining one's life path. In a sense, the two schools are synthesized in Jungian thought, which emphasizes both individuation and the collective unconscious. It is quite common for clients to have some internal conflict themselves regarding their beliefs in this area. Coaches should be aware of their clients' differing beliefs in this area and proceed respectfully. In terms of the pursuit of goals, coaches can help clients achieve a balance between reliance on fate and a belief in total self-determination, while still respecting the clients' spiritual beliefs. In fact, the coach can often use the clients' spiritual or religious beliefs as a framework for articulating goals and a motivating force for pursuing these goals.

Peak Experiences

Often, spirituality can provide the impetus for change, as in the case of peak experiences. A peak experience, according to Maslow, is a moment of epiphany in which an individual feels a rush of excitement and passion about an idea. At this moment, which surpasses ordinary consciousness, everything falls into place and the individual instinctively "knows" what to do. Peak experiences form the highest tier of Maslow's hierarchy of needs and they have the potential to provide enormous motivational power. Because the concept of peak experiences is so powerful as a motivational pull, it is important for coaches to ask their clients if they have had a peak experience and, if so, ask them to describe it. Simply describing their experience can cause them to relive it and can serve to reawaken the motivational feelings or force they once experienced. The peak experience can then be tied in to the client's current motivation struggle and perhaps give some insight into what motivates the client.

Gaining increasing prominence is the belief in the connection between mind, body, and spirit. Two of the most outspoken advocates of the connection among the self-help contingency are Deepak Chopra and Shakti Gawain. Chopra, author of such best-sellers as *The Seven Spiritual Laws of Success* and *Ageless Body, Timeless Mind*, bases his writing in a combination of Eastern and Western philosophy and medicine. He asserts that leading a life of harmony, balance, and spiritual awareness leads to greater health and greater success. Gawain, author of *Creative Visualization*, advocates "creating an inner sanctuary," "opening up the natural energy centers of the body," and using affirmations as tools people can use to achieve their goals and improve their overall health.

Steven Scott similarly advocates a spiritual component of success, although unlike Chopra and Gawain, he does not draw on an Eastern tradition. He writes, "God has given you a mind that is worth far more than [a lot of money]. And it's up to you to be grateful for its endowment, to be excited about learning how to use such a gift to achieve your dreams, and to help others achieve theirs." According to Scott's paradigm, spirituality functions to make one both thankful and confident, both of which contribute to achieving higher levels of motivation.

Positive Affirmations and Self Reinforcement

Affirmations are powerful expressions of thought which many people have found to have amazing impact on realizing one's desires. Beverly Toney-Walter is a writer and personal coach for people who are interested in a spiritual approach to the challenges of personal power, self mastery, and prosperity. She believes that our thoughts create our power. "Manifesting is about the Law of Attraction. Because every thought has creative power, the more you think a thought, the more powerful it becomes. The more passion behind your thought, the more motion goes into the thought and the faster it manifests. In *The Game of Life and How to Play It*, Florence Shinn writes, "Our thoughts, actions and words return to us sooner or later with astounding accuracy. The idea, then, is to think only on what one wants, and not dwell on what one does not want."

Many people ask a "higher power" for their desires to come true. If this has been helpful to the client, then it is useful, and the coach should respectfully incorporate their beliefs into their goals. Such expressions are more common in other cultures and other eras than in present-day America. Nonetheless, an increasing number of self-help books are being written that focus on spirituality. Another idea, less explicitly religious, is for the client to make "grateful" affirmations, such as, "Thank you for giving me the intelligence and skill to succeed in my commercial art business," and "Thank you for bringing me two new clients today." Again, if spirituality or religion inspires the client, this needs to be encouraged.

Toney-Walter believes that our desires are within us for a reason -- a part of a divine plan. Accordingly, in her view, one should not ask for things but give thanks for them and know that one's desire is on its way. In this way, Toney-Walter approaches the issue from a perspective of certitude and trust rather than fear. This theory assumes that what people want is what God and the Universe wants for them. Coaches need to respect the spiritual belief system of the client while providing a supportive environment in which desired change can occur.

Visualizations

Interventions such as guided imagery, visualizations, and hypnosis have shown to be very effective in motivational training. The "vision" (or image) one might create is how one's life will look when he/she has achieved one's goals. One could also create the vision of performing well at a desired skill. There can be many "visions" representing different aspects, or stages of the goal. The coach can assist clients in creating a "vision" (as described in a previous chapter) that they can "go to" at any time they need reinforcement. Another, more concrete method of using visualizations, is to have clients put pictures that represent their "vision" in conspicuous places around their home, car, appointment book, etc. When one saturates oneself with their vision of their goal attainment, it can help motivate and keep them on track.

In sports motivation, Richard Suinn, Ph.D., sports psychologist, teaches his clients skills such as stress management, self-regulation, visualization, goal-setting, concentration, focus, and even relaxation. He has written about a technique he calls "mental practice," which is also referred to as "visualization" or "imagery rehearsal." "It's the mental equivalent of physical practice," says Suinn. There is research evidence that indicates that when athletes use visualization after relaxation, their performance improves. The converse also holds true, if they imagine themselves doing poorly their performance worsens.

Your Words are Your Power

Your word is the power you have to create. Your word is the power you have to motivate yourself. Words can literally change our beings and actions. In her book, *The Right Words at the Right Time*, Marlo Thomas provides a wonderful expose of the words that motivated a variety of people who have achieved great things. She discusses how words have a tremendous impact on us. They can either serve to move us to action or to keep us down. For example, she quotes:

"Muhammad Ali responded to a teacher's assertion that he 'ain't never gonna be nuthin'. Billy Crystal, Walter Cronkite, Katie Couric and Kenneth Cole also received words of discouragement that

goaded them on to achievement. The right words
moved Al Pacino to pull out of a downward spiral.
Paul McCartney's words came in a dream; Steven
Spielberg's came from Davey Crockett. Chris
Rock's words, like mine, came from his father;
Supreme Court Justice Ruth Bader Ginsburg's from
her mother-in-law on the eve of her wedding.
Rudolph Giuliani, Cindy Crawford and Gwyneth
Paltrow heard the words that changed their lives
during a moment of crisis."

Some positive self-statements come to us
naturally, and some are much more difficult to fuse
into our being. One of the words I often use is
"intention." Intention is what we want to have
happen – our primary objective – our true aim. When
I wake up in the morning I think about how I want
my day to go. I say "My intention today is to be safe,
happy and healthy, and to complete one chapter in
my book." My day usually goes according to my
intention. However, sometimes it seems the whole
world is conspiring against my intention. Lots of
distractions come up, people don't do what they are
supposed to do, things are delayed for reasons
beyond my control, things break down and I have to
stop and fix them, etc. I have to be flexible and
patient during these times.

Usually however, what stops my intentions is
my own refusal to set limits with others. People
distract me and get me off my course by either asking
for my help, or attempting to engage me in THEIR
problems/crises/dramas. This is where I am weakest,
as I am by nature a people-helper. So what I have
learned to do (when possible) is to tell (not ask)
others what my intentions are, and that after my
intentions have been met, I will be available to them.
By the time I'm ready for them, they have usually
solved their own problem!

Sometimes, with certain people, I have to change the word "intend" to "insist." Sometimes it's okay to insist that things go your way. As long as you are not stepping on anyone else's toes, or harming anyone else, or neglecting to care for those who really need you, you have the right to insist on doing your own thing, i.e. getting to your appointment on time or completing your goal on time.

Reward yourself with your words. Praise yourself for a job well-done, or a step on your plan completed. For example, if you have just accomplished something that was a challenge for you, pat yourself on the back and say "Wow, that really took perseverance, but I did it." It is very important to remind yourself often of how far you've come in your journey.

Life is a rush into the unknown.
You can duck down and hope nothing hits you, or
stand up tall as you can, show it your teeth and say
"Bring it on, Baby, and don't be stingy with the
jalapenos!"
---Anonymous

Chapter Eleven:
Keeping Clients in Coaching Until
Goals are Accomplished

The best coaches really care about people. They have a sincere interest in people.
---Byron & Catherine Pulsifer, from *What Are People's Expectations of a Coach?*

Because keeping clients in a coaching program is a prerequisite to implementing the rest of the motivational techniques and strategies described in this book, this chapter serves as both an introduction to the rest of the book and also a summary of it -- a good place for readers to begin and to end. As a result, many of the ideas from other chapters are referred to and at times even summarized in this chapter. These inclusions are intended to refresh the memories of those who have already read the preceding chapters and to refer those who haven't yet read other chapters to those chapters that will be most useful to them personally.

Hidden Reasons Clients Quit a Program Too Soon

According to James Prochaska's research, clients quit treatment too soon 45% of the time. Only 9% state "fees" as the reason. An overwhelming 68% state "an attitude of indifference on the part of the caregiver." Therefore, it is extremely important for coaches to use humanistic approaches with clients, such as unconditional positive regard, empathic responses, active listening, and a sense of genuine warmth.

The coach can get an idea of how long a client will remain in coaching by finding out how long the client has stayed in a program in a prior course (a "course" refers to a sequence of sessions of coaching or treatment). Clients usually follow patterns of behavior. If this person has not been in coaching at a prior time, the coach can at least find out how long they have stayed in other courses, such as medical treatment, dental treatment, self-help courses, educational classes, training courses, and relationships. In his book *The Bipersonal Field*, Robert Langs discusses the concept of de-coding unconscious messages. He explains that one can tell how long a person will commit to a program by their stories about prior activities. The coach can ascertain clients' patterns and relate those patterns to their current course of sessions. The goal, states Langs, is to make these patterns conscious to the client and to assist him/her in first making the change here, in this program, by staying with it for a specified period of time. This will be the first step in assisting the client in changing his/her pattern of quitting too soon.

"Too soon" can be defined as any time at which clients have not yet received the greatest value from their sessions and have not yet implemented positive changes over a long enough period of time to change habits in a lasting way. The amount of time this takes is ultimately up to the client to decide, since remaining in coaching is always the client's choice.

Clients end a program too soon for many reasons. Most clients will give a reason for quitting, but their stated reason often masks other underlying reasons. Coaches have a responsibility to attempt to understand the real reasons their clients quit a program prior to completion. Finding out the real reason can be a challenge, as you must respect your clients' privacy and confidentiality. One very successful way to uncover the unstated reasons is to mail out a <u>Client Satisfaction Questionnaire</u> to all former clients. The clients do not need to put their names on it, so that they can be completely honest. Include a self-addressed, stamped envelope for quick reply. This will give you an idea of how you are doing from the clients' point of view and will reveal whether a client left because of dissatisfaction. You can then know what improvements you need to effect in order to be a better coach. I recommend giving clients a satisfaction survey to complete after every 3 or 4 sessions. This way you can intercept potential problems before they have a chance to develop. Questionnaires also give clients a forum to voice any complaints they may have without the embarrassment of face-to-face confrontation. Finally, questionnaires give clients the feeling that their coach cares about them and conducts a practice with responsibility and a desire for improvement.

    <u>One reason</u> clients quit too soon may be that they are <u>unhappy with the service</u> they are receiving, as explained above. <u>Another reason</u> may be that they <u>do not feel there is a good "fit" or connection</u> between themselves and their coach. This may also be brought out in the satisfaction questionnaire, and the coach should not take such comments personally. We cannot be all things to all people. If the coach becomes aware of a lack of connection as a reason for the client wishing to leave coaching, the coach should make every effort to refer the client to another coach with whom there may be a better fit. However, if there seems to be a pattern of feedback regarding connection or joining, particularly if clients often state something like "the coach didn't seem to understand me," this is cause for concern. The coach would then be wise to get some training in this area from a supervisor, colleagues, or at a workshop or class.

A <u>third reason</u> clients may quit before they have met their desired goals is that they are <u>resistant to change</u> or the work involved in changing has become too difficult. A perceptive coach will pick up on these cues before the client quits and will attempt to work through them with the person. The most difficult aspect of motivation is that of persistence. How does the coach assist the client in developing this quality? One way, as I have pointed out, is to help the client keep his/her sight on the goal and remind him/her of how good it will feel to have achieved it. Perhaps the one, most common way that coaches fail to keep clients in a program is that they do not educate their clients about the rocky road ahead. An effective coach will predict the difficulties that will come (sabotages, blocks, setbacks, etc.) and assist the client in planning and preparing themselves mentally for these obstacles. When a client begins to lose interest or motivation, the coach needs to address this as an important issue, so that the client does not view the coach as apathetic or ambivalent. If clients see their coach as having a laissez-faire attitude, it will be easier for them to quit and they will feel justified in doing so. The concepts of commitment, determination, and persistence are explained in Chapter 6, "Thought Transformation." This chapter is extremely useful in helping the coach to assist clients in setting goals, keeping commitments, and staying on track. On the other hand, coaches must be careful never to push or dominate clients to continue with a program, as their participation is completely their choice.

A <u>fourth</u>, common reason clients give for leaving a program early is that they <u>cannot afford to continue</u>. This may be a reality, and it is an issue that all coaches and coaches face in their practices. I do not generally recommend decreasing fees, as this can set up a dependency situation (both ways), or a problematic boundary situation. If, however, the client's inability to pay appears to be sincere (recent job loss, financial setback, etc.), and his/her desire to continue a program is sincere, the coach should use judgment in decreasing fees on a temporary basis. Alternatively, sessions can be held less frequently. It may also be a reality that the client can afford it but does not view the benefits received as being worth the fee. In this case, decreasing fees would only serve to weaken the perceived value of the service. In any case, if the client states that he/she cannot afford the fee, and the coach does not wish to negotiate, it is crucial that the coach respect this and offer several referral sources where the client can be assisted at a lower fee.

Despite the emphasis on keeping clients in a program until goals have been met, coaches must give clients permission to stop their process, even stop their program, at any time they choose (with at least 24 hours notice, of course). Let them know that clients often stop coming to treatment/coaching when the road gets too rough, and that it is acceptable to take a break, and it is acceptable to return later. Many times clients will feel like quitting but will remember your having said that this feeling is normal and to be expected. This may help them to press on, knowing it is a challenge they need to overcome. If the client insists on terminating before you feel they are ready, discuss with the client ways to recognize signs of re-occurrence and ways to cope with the problem should they recur.

It is also important to let clients know that taking a break from coaching is acceptable, because an extremely common scenario is that clients will stop a program before they have attained their goals and later, in a few weeks, or a few months, they will want to return. However, often they are too embarrassed to call their coach and ask for an appointment because they feel they let their coach down. This feeling of having "let you down" will serve as a motivation blocker and may actually weigh on the client's psyche for years. Predicting this scenario, and giving clients permission to return at any time without remorse or embarrassment, will assist them in getting back on track towards their goals and continuing with their process much more quickly.

If you have been in practice for a while, you can probably think of many clients who quit their program too soon. Many of your former clients can be reactivated (motivated to return to treatment or coaching), if you do one simple thing -- send them a reactivation letter. This is an invitation to come back to treatment or to accomplish further goals if they wish. It tells them you care about their treatment and that you would be happy to work with them again. At best, it will cause them to return to work with you. At worst, it allows them to "save face" with you and frees them from the heavy burden of feeling they let you down. So it is a "win-win" situation.

Sample Reactivation Letter

Dear Client:

How are you doing? It's been a while since I've seen you. I am writing this letter for several reasons. First, I want you to know I hope you are doing well. Second, I want you to know I've made some changes at the office. I have completed a certification program and am a "Certified Professional Coach" in addition to being a coach. I am now able to assist people with attaining goals for a more satisfied life experience. I have also added a new partner. Her name is Susan Morrow, Ph.D., and she specializes in children's learning disorders. We also have a new receptionist, Becky Smith, who will answer phones and greet clients daily from noon to 8 P.M. Feel free to call her (or my voice mail) if you would like to set up an appointment. I would be happy to assess the goals you have for your future. Third, I would greatly appreciate it if you would take a few minutes to complete the enclosed "Client Satisfaction Survey." This is the best way I know to find out how I can improve my skills. You do not have to put your name on it, so you can feel free to be honest.

Again, I hope this letter finds you well. Sincerely,

Jill Cohen, Ph.D.

Program Structure

One of the first steps in the coaching process is to have the coach and client agree upon the structure of the program: length of sessions, frequency of sessions, projected length of the program. The most important first question the coach needs to ask his/her client is, "How will you know when it is time to stop coming?" Use the answer to this question as a guidepost when assessing or re-assessing how long the program should be. As an example, see the guidelines described in my e-book, *How to Become a Personal Coach"* in which I recommend beginning with a minimum amount of time, a 12-week course, one hour per week. Clients do want to know <u>how</u> you will help them, and approximately how long it will take. This will educate them prior to beginning the course, so that they can give informed consent.

The strategies for structuring a program are applicable to consulting and training work with businesses and corporations as well as to a individual coaching program. Coaching is now recognized within the corporate culture as <u>more positive, effective, and empowering than instruction</u>. It is a vital force in motivating employees. There is a great deal of support from corporate executives for motivational programs. Supervisors and managers would benefit from learning how to motivate their staff as well as themselves. Career coaching is one of the fastest growing niches in the counseling profession. When providing career coaching with individuals and corporations, the same program structure described here needs to be followed. A 12-week program, is recommended, however, a short, introductory class may be helpful to get the participants to "buy in" to a full program. During the introduction, it is important to educate the prospective clients about the program structure. Provide an outline like the one given in my e-book *How to Become a Personal Coach.*

There will be many times that clients will not feel particularly intrinsically motivated to come to their sessions and would therefore be tempted not to show had they not paid in advance and made a commitment to the program. This scenario can be used as a metaphor for the difficult work that clients encounter while struggling to stay on their course toward their goals. An effective coach will point this out during each session and validate client's continuance, especially when the work is difficult.

Program Goals

Most clients who enter a coaching program will be in need of assistance in the decision making process. It is amazing how many coaches will go on and on with the client, for months or even years, without ever providing their clients with a basic structure for the decision-making process. People who are indecisive need structure, rules, lists and organization. It is the responsibility of the coach to provide this. Here is a list of the components of the basic decision-making process:

1.List your personal values and prioritize them.

2.List your options (the coach can brainstorm with the client).
3.Write the possible outcomes for each option.
4.Get more information about the possible outcomes.
5.Write the pros and cons for each option.
6.Talk with experts about the options.
7.Talk with 3 supportive/trusted people about the options.
8.Determine which option corresponds most closely with your values.
9.Determine which option is the healthiest for all involved.
10.Make a decision that you can commit to for a specified period of time.
11.Re-evaluate and/or make changes after the specified period of time.

Once the decision has been made by the client regarding his/her goals, it is important for the coach and client to assess the "healthiness" of these goals in the overall context of the client's life. Chapter 2, "Assessing Healthy and Unhealthy Goals," discusses information that is critical to assisting clients in determining healthy goals. In his book *8 Weeks to Optimum Health*, Andrew Weil discusses the importance of having a healthy balance in the physical, mental, spiritual, and emotional realms. It is important that all of these areas are taken into full consideration when defining goals.

The coach can assist the client in setting appropriate, attainable goals, and once the desired goals have been settled upon, they can be put down in writing. Structuring a "Goals Process" is often omitted from ongoing, long-term sessions, yet it is a crucial component of motivation and success. This process is outlined and explained more fully in Chapter 8, "Goal Setting," but the basic 5-step process is as follows:

1) Define your vision or mission statement in writing.
2) Convert your vision into specific goals.
3) Convert each goal into specific steps.
4) Convert each step into specific tasks.
5) Assign a projected time or date to complete each task.

These structures may seem trivial or elementary to the clinician, who has already achieved many goals related to education and training. Yet for many clients, these steps are not obvious. Moreover, lower functioning clients may have difficulty making decisions, let alone setting goals or following through on commitments. There is a tendency for some coaches to want to say to their clients, "ENOUGH ALREADY! JUST DO IT!!" Working with clients to set goals and then meet them can admittedly be frustrating work. Chapter 12, "Motivation for the Mental Health Provider," assists clinicians with these difficult points in their careers. The most important thing to remember is that most clients never got these "simple life instructions" prior to visiting their coach. This may be the only place they can ever get this kind of valuable education. You went into this field to make a difference in the quality of people's lives, and the area of motivation is one in which you can make a big difference.

The role of the coach in motivational coaching is to be a facilitator and guide, one who assists clients in setting goals and then helps them measure their progress. Thus, the coach and the client need to agree upon a few stated goals that can be measured objectively. For example, "When I can relax" is not sufficient. A more specific measure might be broken down into several parts: "When I am able to determine immediately whether the actions of those around me are life threatening to me or not;" "When those actions are not life threatening, I will be able to respond calmly, in a tone of voice no higher than a 5 (on a scale of 1 - 10);" and "When my blood pressure goes down below 180 and is sustained for over a period of three months." It is very beneficial to a client's motivation to measure (in writing, in the form of an action plan) the amount of work he or she has done and then mark the work as completed on the time plan, since this demonstrates that progress is being made. When a goal is marked as completed, the client will be more motivated to start the next one.

Program Support

As explained in Chapter Three, "Comparison of Professional and Self-help Literature," outcome studies are the best evidence of what works and what does not in the area of effecting life change. Therefore, you can be more influential as a coach if you quote outcome studies to your clients or, better yet, hand them copies of the articles themselves. This means that you must be in the business of keeping up with professional literature, which is time consuming. But if you are specializing in one to three areas of expertise, reading one research study a week should not be that difficult. Plan on putting at least one to two hours per week into studying new psychological research. It will prove worthwhile when your client is motivated by the fact that something has been proven to work for the majority of people.

Testimonials and anecdotes, which are easily found in self-help literature, and which you can encourage your clients to seek out or which you can share with them during sessions, can further inspire clients. For example, "rags-to-riches" stories abound: people who came from poor, unfortunate circumstances and rose above them because of determination and will. Relating these stories to clients is an excellent way to assist them in working through their blocks as well as inspiring them. The reason this strategy works so well is that people learn easily from imitation. Having as a model a person who has undergone similar struggles and has overcome them is an effective way to inspire change.

An extensive amount of research has been done in the fields of weight loss and drug/alcohol cessation to determine what motivates people to change habits when they are reluctant to do so. The results overwhelmingly indicate the influence of personal interaction on a regular basis with a support person(s) who understands the problem and will encourage, support, validate and inspire change. The number one method of personal support is face-to-face individual and/or group meetings. If the coach has a large enough clientele to warrant a group, it is extremely beneficial to offer this service in addition to individual sessions. Many clients cannot afford individual coaching; moreover, as a client who has been in an individual program gets toward the end of a course of the program, he or she can be transferred into a group which will provide ongoing support. The work of Abraham Maslow, the great humanistic psychologist, correlates with the findings of the above-mentioned research on the value of personal support. Maslow believed that a person would move themselves up the "hierarchy of needs" ladder naturally, as each previous need was satisfied. Consequently, he viewed the coach's role as primarily one of support, encouragement, and positive regard. If you are interested in becoming a weight control or fitness coach, read my e-book *How to Stick With Your Diet and Exercise Program.*

The Best Motivational Strategies

Coaches are often models for their clients as well as support figures. <u>Who</u> you are as a coach is often at least as important as <u>what</u> you do. Your clients (hopefully) look up to you as a highly educated and experienced person in the area of life with which they have hired you to assist them. Many of them will view you as a role model or mentor as well as a teacher and counselor. Because of this, it is important for you to appear professional and confident yet also warm and caring.

Think for a moment about what you have done in your life, what you have accomplished and the motivation required to reach the goals you have met. In order to become a coach, you had to complete assignments, pass tests, write papers, pass courses, take entrance exams, get college degrees, complete internships, get supervised work experience, perhaps write a dissertation, take licensing exams, etc. You did all this, while also doing other important things, like working, taking care of children, being a lover or spouse, taking care of a home, exercising, pursuing hobbies, and engaging in other social and professional activities. This is a huge achievement! And right now you are probably working on new goals for yourself such as becoming a motivational coach.

Take the time to write out your story, not for your clients but for yourself. This will enable you to process internally how you achieved many of your own goals. You will carry with you a sense of confidence that comes from mastery and this will show up in your work with clients. There is no need to disclose your story to your clients, however, you may want to use bits and pieces of it along the way if you feel it is relevant to a client's situation and enhances their motivational process. There is much more information regarding this topic specifically for the coach in Chapter 12, "Motivation for the Mental Health Provider."

A powerful strategy to motivate clients, developed by Thomas J. Leonard, is called "What I want for you is . . ." If it is used sparingly and is well placed, it can act as a great motivator. The strategy simply involves telling the client what you would like for him or her. It cannot be argued with. Expressing these ambitions and dreams makes clients feel that you care about them and want something good for them. As a result, they will listen to what you say and feel motivated to act in a manner that will facilitate the actualization of your statement. The following are some generic examples of what a coach might want for their clients:

--What I want for you is for you to look out for your best interests and take care of yourself.
--What I want for you is for you to consider the impact of your actions on your children.
--What I want for you is for you to decide on some concrete ways to decrease your stress.
--What I want for you is for you to be a positive, productive, contributing member of society.
--What I want for you is for you to gain skills that will make you feel better about yourself.
--What I want for you is for you to have only healthy, supportive people around you.
--What I want for you is for you to achieve this goal as soon as possible.

Make a list of at least three "What I want for you" statements for each of your existing clients. This will help you to review your clients' basic issues and find the words and language you need to express these wishes at the optimal time.

There is one thing you can do as a coach-motivator that can cause you to be more influential with your clients. It is a skill that self-help writer Barbara De Angelis developed and it has caused her to be enormously influential. You can begin to get a feel for it when you read her career goals. She states, "I never wanted to be famous, but I did want to be influential. I know I've been sent here for a reason.

I'm not the most brilliant thinker in the world or the most original, but I really understand communication. I think I know how to take important concepts and ideas and reach people and touch them. I want to touch as many people as I can and open their hearts to love so that, hopefully, at the end of my life there will be millions of people who are living much more loving lives because of whatever I did."

De Angelis uses the gift of <u>passion</u>. Passion is communicated when others can feel the importance that you place on what you are saying. If you as a coach believe that a certain concept is extremely important to the well-being of your clients, you need to communicate it in a way that they will feel it. Your feelings of passion can be contagious, which is how Anthony Robbins gets more than 5,000 people to attend his seminars. When people walk away from hearing a positive and influential speaker, they may be thinking, "That person was a great speaker," but hopefully they are also thinking, "I feel great."

Here is GROW's simple 5 step coaching process -- you can do this exercise with anyone, anywhere, in as little as 10 minutes:

1) What do you want? (Formulate the goal in a sentence with a noun, a verb, and a time to complete)
2) What can you do this week toward your goal?
3) What might stop you?
4) How will you overcome it?
5) When will you let me know you've completed it?

<u>Encouraging Clients to Show Up for Their Next Scheduled Visit</u>

I have found that there are some specific things coaches can say at the end of each session to increase the likelihood that their clients will show up for their next scheduled visit. Referring back to the first part of this chapter, remember that the most important thing coaches can do is to provide structure for their clients. I recommend you follow this guide:

1) Assess with the client where you currently are in the program structure. For example, "You've just completed session #4 and next week we will begin session #5--We'll be discussing the obstacles that could hinder your progress and how to overcome them." This statement tells the client that he/she has completed another program goal, which produces a feeling of success. It also communicates that the client is still in the middle of a process, which motivates him/her to continue to complete the steps leading up to the realization of his/her final goal.

2) Give the client a homework assignment to return the following week. This can be one or two of the worksheets in the *Client Motivation Workbook* or something else that you and your client have agreed upon. Homework assignments encourage clients to show up for their next visit, as they will want your feedback on their work. Try to make sure the assignment is not too overwhelming, because if they do not complete it, clients may have reservations about showing up for their next scheduled visit for fear of disappointing you. For this reason, make sure you tell clients, "Don't worry if you don't finish this, since we can then work on it during our next session."

3) It is crucial that at the end of each session you validate your clients on the progress they have made on their goals. Show them their "Goals Ladder" that you have already created, and point out where they are on it. For example, "Last week you were here and now you are here. You've made visible progress this week. Congratulations." Again, let them know that if they did not make progress this week, such delays and setbacks are part of the normal process and provide an opportunity to analyze and overcome any obstacles that might have come up.

4) Remind your clients of their goals for the next week and give them a supportive and encouraging statement such as, "You stated that your plan for this next week is to obtain at least 3 applications from graduate programs. I'm excited about you taking this next step in your goal process." This simple statement instills motivation and increases the likelihood that your clients will show up for their next visit.

To increase the likelihood that your clients will show up for their next scheduled visit, I recommend that you <u>give them three things</u> prior to their leaving the current session:

1) An appointment card with your "no-show" policy on it
2) A homework assignment
3) An affirmation for the week

<u>Ending a Coaching Program</u>

Generally, at some point during the course of the program, clients will have a sense that they have been helped enough or have received what they can from the course and now can continue making progress on their own. If you and your client have been following the program structure outlined in the supplemental *How to Become a Personal Coach,* it will be very clear when termination is approaching. This is the point to begin discussing a "phasing out" process, which can mean less frequent sessions, a temporary hiatus, or termination planning. Through this process, the client and coach can assess the readiness of the client to end his/her sessions. It is important to let clients know that just because this phase of the program is ending, it does not mean that goal setting itself ends. There may be more work for clients to do on their own or through another course, and there may be a point in the future when clients desire to re-enter a new goal attainment program with you. Let your clients know that it is acceptable to you to take a break and renew the program at a later date. Many goals are lifetime projects and successive courses of update sessions are an ideal way of keeping track of progress.

While the ending point in a course of coaching or treatment is ultimately determined by the client, it ideally will be a joint agreement by coach and client. The most effective way to keep retain client's motivation until they have achieved their goals is to provide <u>excellent service</u>. This means assessing, structuring, guiding, supporting, encouraging, motivating and inspiring positive personal change. I hope I have provided more education and tools for you to succeed as an effective motivator of change in the coaching and/or change process.

*Executives and HR managers know coaching is the most potent tool
for inducing lasting personal change.*
---Ivy Business Journal

Chapter Twelve:
Motivation for Coaches and Helping Professionals

Make no mistake, as you change your leadership style to one of a coach you will face challenges. There will be times when you question why am I doing this. However, you must at all times keep the long term benefits of being a coach at the forefront of your mind.
---Byron & Catherine Pulsifer, from *Challenges in Adopting a Coaching Style*

Remaining consistently motivated is difficult in any profession. It is particularly difficult in the helping professions, such as teaching, nursing, and psychology. People who enter these professions are usually idealistic and aspire to help others in profound ways. Thus, their guilt, frustration and sense of failure are particularly acute when they find themselves unable to meet the expectations and demands they have set for themselves. In the mental health field, the risk of burnout is especially high because the work is so emotionally draining. Treatment involves an inevitable lack of reciprocity: the coach gives and the client takes. Coaches are emotionally taxed by working with people suffering from depression and related problems. They are further frustrated by working with clients who seem to make no progress or who expect the coach to "cure" them or "fix" their problems. Moreover, coaches are rarely given the chance to enjoy their clients' improvement, since when the clients feel that their problems are under control, they usually leave treatment.

Preventing Caregiver Burnout

Finding a support system to combat burnout is difficult for coaches. They usually work in isolation and then are bound by confidentiality not to discuss clients with friends and family. This tends to make coaches both professionally and personally isolated. Yet coaches often fail to realize the factors that contribute to their own stress, depression, isolation, and burnout. Because mental health professionals are trained to focus on and analyze the needs of their clients, they tend to overlook their own needs.

The current climate of managed care takeovers adds an additional source of stress: Fees are lower, longer hours are dedicated to paperwork, remaining time and energy are devoted to establishing phone contact with third-party reimbursers, etc. It used to be that indemnity insurance paid 80% of whatever the charges were, no questions asked! To add to these difficulties, the current market is over-saturated. There are too many coaches, the climate is more competitive, and coaches are not trained to excel in competitive situations or to negotiate complicated bureaucratic transactions.

These factors together conspire to give coaches feelings of powerlessness and lack of control over work and income. So what can be done to remain motivated and successful in this environment?

Operating at Peak Performance

Kilburg, Nathan, and Thoreson described a continuum along which professional performance operates:

--Peak
--Normal
--Distressed/impaired

--Burned out
--Disabled

Consider where you would place yourself on this continuum. Because of the number of factors which contribute to burnout, most coaches are not able to assert confidently that they are operating according to their "peak" performance. According to Maslach, "distress" includes emotional exhaustion, depersonalization, and reduced sense of personal accomplishment. Working at a lower level than this implies a risk to your own professional responsibilities and to your clients' well being. One of the worst effects of burnout is poor judgment. When coaches suffer from poor judgment, they are no longer able to make the best choices for themselves and their clients and, as a result, their level of burnout escalates. Similarly, although isolation is one of the causes of burnout, people who suffer from burnout tend to isolate themselves further and to drive potential supporters away by behaving in hostile and overly cynical ways (Cherniss, *The Burnout Syndrome*).

Recognizing signs of burnout is one of the first steps to combating it. For example, if you can tell that you are functioning at a "distressed level," you can make sure that your work never deteriorates to the "impaired" level. In *Toxic Burnout*, which stresses a mind-body connection, Barbara Reinhold asserts that the body sends alert signals when burnout begins, and that if one can learn to recognize these bodily signs, one can intervene and burnout can be averted. Coaches are bound ethically and legally to function responsibly and professionally. Therefore, they must <u>continually engage in self-evaluation and self-regulation</u> so as to avoid the pitfalls of burnout.

There is hope for avoiding burnout. Other coaches have found ways to avoid burnout and become more motivated, and so can you.

Furthermore, a burnout crisis can stimulate introspection and analysis and thereby serve as an impetus for new professional and personal growth.

If you are interested in learning more about self-motivation and burn-out prevention for coaches, read my e-book *Seven Secrets of Highly Successful Therapists*. This book will teach you the primary strategies for remaining motivated, challenged, and satisfied in the mental health profession:

--How to change your work environment so as to reduce stress and increase motivation.
--How to avoid the pitfalls of self-blame.
--New ways to make your job more satisfying, including suggestions for ways to diversify your routine and tips on the hottest new areas of specialization.
--Strategies for increasing your support network.
--How to identify alternative income sources.
--Suggestions for ways to challenge yourself and become more professionally engaged.
--Strategies for balancing career and personal development.

Coaches are not immune from the problems they help their clients work through, but because helping professionals are taught to focus on their clients, they often neglect their own problems. By devoting time to your own motivational process, you will achieve your career dreams and will be a better coach as a result. The more professionally motivated you are, the more your clients will pick up on this energy and become motivated themselves. The more excited you are about your work, the more you have to give to your clients.

Nothing motivates like success. When people work in a supportive and challenging environment, they can work to the height of their potential; their resulting success then strengthens their initial motivation, creating a positive cycle. However, it is up to you to follow a motivational program, put it into practice, and initiate this cycle.

<u>The 7-Step Success Cycle</u>

1.Give gratitude
2.Intent, purpose and goals -- and go get it!
3.Have patience, endure short term discomfort
4.Receive it!
5.Maintain it -- take care of it!
6.Protect it -- if you don't, you won't keep it!
7.Give gratitude (starts the process over again for your next new and great goal!

Thank you for reading this book. May you get motivated, stay motivated, and find people in your life to help motivate you. May you motivate others to do more than they thought they could. May you rise to your full potential and experience fabulous success!

Every calling is great when greatly pursued.
---Oliver Wendell Holmes, Jr.

Bibliography

Bandura, Albert. (1977) *Social learning theory.* Englewood Cliffs, NJ: Prentice Hall.

Biography magazine. (1998 - 2005) Various articles on specific high achievers. Jan - Dec, 1998.

Bliss, Edwin. (1986) *Doing it now.* New York: Simon & Schuster.

Borysenko, J. (2001) *Fire in the soul.*

Braham, Barbara. (2009) *Finding Your Purpose.* Crisp Publications, Menlo Park, CA.

Breathnach, Sarah. (1995) *Simple abundance.* New York: Warner Books.

Brounstein, Marty. (2001) *Coaching & mentoring for dummies.* IDG Books. New York, NY.

Brown, Les. 1992. *Live your dreams.* Avon Books, Inc. New York, NY.

Chopra, Deepak, MD. (1995) *The seven spiritual laws of success.* Amber-Allen.

Deci, Edward L. (1985) *Intrinsic motivation and self-determination in human behavior.* New York: Plenum.

Dyer, Wayne. (1980) *The sky's the limit.* New York: Pocket Books.

Epstein, Robert, Ph.D. (1999) Helping athletes go for the gold. *Psychology Today.* May/June, 1999, p.20.

Feinbert, M. (1992) Why smart people do dumb things. *Wall Street Journal*. Dec. 21, 1992. New York, NY.

Fowler, S. (2014) Why motivating people doesn't work and what does: The new science of leading, energizing, and engaging.

Gawain, Shakti. (1995) *Creative visualization*. San Rafael, CA: New World Library.

Goleman, D. (2002) Could you be a leader? *Parade Magazine*. June 16.

Heller, Sharon, Ph.D. (1999) *The complete idiot's guide to conquering fear and anxiety*. Alpha Books. New York, NY.

Hennessey, Beth A, & Amabile, Teresa M. (1998) Reality, intrinsic motivation, and creativity. *American Psychologist*. P. 53, 674-675.

Hill, Napolean, (1990) *Think and grow rich*. New York: Doubleday.

Hudson, Frederic M. (1999) *The handbook of coaching*. CA: Jossey-Bass Publishers.

Hukill, Traci, (1999) Mentoring for the 90's. *Family Therapy Networker*. May/June 1999.

Isaacs, Ernest. (1997) Taming the inner critic. *The California Coach*. Sept./Oct. 1997.

Kelley, Lyn. Is it okay to want to help people and make money too? *The Coach*, CAAMFT. July/Aug. 2005.

-----. Motivating clients to show up for their next scheduled visit. *Counseling Today*, ACA. Aug. 2006.

-----. Coach to coach: ethical considerations. *Family Therapy News*. Apr/May 2000.

-----. *How to Become a Personal Coach, How to Become Your Own Life Coach, How to Become a Virtual Coach, How to Become a Corporate or Business Coach, How to Motivate People! The 3 Magic Keys to Unlocking Anyone's Hidden Motivation, How to Stick With Your Diet and Exercise Program.*

Leonard, Thomas J. (1998) *The portable coach.* NY: Soribner.

Lerner, Mary Ellin. Goodbye couch. Hello, coach. *USA Weekend.* Lifestyles section. March 2001.

Maslach, C., Jackson, S.E., and Leitner, M.P. (1996) *Maslach burnout inventory manual.* (3d edition). Consulting Psychologists Press.

Maslow, Abraham. (1970) *Motivation and personality.* (2nd ed.). New York: Harper and Row.

McClelland, David C. (1985) *Human motivation.* Glenview, Ill.: Scott, Foresman.

Mc Graw, Phil. (1999) *Life strategies.* Hyperion: New York, NY.

Menendez, D. and Williams, P. (2018) Becoming a professional life coach: Lessons from the Institute of Life Coach Training.

Miller, J. (2018) How to motivate people: Little known secrets you need to know.

Millman, Dan. (2001) *Living on purpose.* New World Library: Novato, CA.

O'Neil, Harold F., & Drillings, Michael. (Eds.). (1994) *Motivation: theory and research.* Hillsdale, NJ: L. Erlbaum Associates.

Prochaska, J.O., Norcross, J.C., and DiClimente, C.C. (1997) *Changing for good.* New York: Avon.

Robbins, Anthony. (2011) *Unlimited power.* New York: Fawcett Books.

Roger, John & McWilliams, Peter. (1991) *Do it! Let's get off our bu*ts. Los Angeles: Prelude Press.

Rothman, Smith, Nakashima, Paterson, and Mustin. (1996) Client self-determination and professional intervention. *Social Work.* 41:4.

Scott, Steven K. (1998) *Simple steps to impossible dreams.* New York: Simon and Schuster.

Seligman, Martin E.P. (1994) *What you can change and what you can't.* New York: A.A. Knopf

----. (1997) *Learned Helplessness..* New York: A.A. Knopf.

Sheehy, Gail. (1985) *Passages.* New York: Bantam.

-----. (1981) *Pathfinders.* New York: Bantam.

Sher, Barbara. (1994) *I could be anything if only I knew what it was.* NY: Delacorte.

-----. (2001) *It's never too late unless you don't start now.*

Shinn, Florence. (1980) *The game of life and how to play it.* New York: Simon and Schuster.

Stecker, T. (2011) Using a brief intervention to motivate clients to get help: A how to manual for professionals.

Twerski, Abraham. (1997) *Life's too short!* New York: St. Martin's Griffin.

Viorst, Judith. (1998) *Imperfect control.* New York: Simon and Schuster.

Waitley, Denis. (2007) *The new dynamics of goal setting.* New York: William Morrow.

Warren, Rick. (2002) *The purpose driven life.* Zondervan: Grand Rapids, MI.

Weinschen, S. (2013) How to get people to do stuff: Master the art and science of persuasion and motivation.

Williams, Patrick. (2007) Becoming a professional life coach. W.W. Norton and Co., Inc. New York, NY.

-----. (2022) *Therapist as life coach.* Norton: New York, NY.

###

Discover other titles by Lyn Kelley distributed at
<u>www.Amazon.com</u>

<u>New Release!</u>
Bad Dick, Good Jane: How Good Girls Get Bad Boys to Behave

<u>Dear Jane Series:</u>
The 12 Biggest Mistakes Women Make in Dating & Love Relationships
How to Turn a Player into a Stayer
How to Cure a Commitment-Phobic
Controlling and Manipulative Men: How to Spot Them and Handle Them
Self-Centered and Narcissistic Men: How to Spot Them and Handle Them
Addicted Men: How to Spot Them and Handle Them
Low Achieving Men - Passives, Wimps, Dreamers: How to Spot Them and Handle Them
Cheap Men: How to Spot Them and Handle Them
Men who Lie and Cheat: How to Spot Them and Handle Them
Emotionally Unavailable Men: How to Spot Them and Handle Them
10 Secrets to Getting Any Man You Want to Want YOU
How to Break Up, Survive and Thrive

How to Stick With Your Diet & Exercise Program
How to Motivate People! The 3 Magic Keys to Unlock Anyone's Hidden Motivation
Therapists: How to Promote Your Practice to a Well-Pay, Self-Pay Clientele
Healthcare Providers: How to Promote Your Practice to a Well-Pay, Self-Pay Clientele

How to Motivate Your Clients to Change:
Psychological Principles of Motivation
How to Become a Life Coach
How to Become a Corporate/Business Coach
How to Become a Virtual Coach
The 7 Secrets of Highly Successful Therapists
The 7 Self-Sabotages: Why People Sabotage
Themselves and How to Stop It
Alternative Income Sources for Therapists
Ethical Issues for Coaches
Practice Angels: How to Build a Full Practice from
Good Referral Sources Alone
How to Get a Raise from Managed Care Plans
Get New Clients Now! Top 10 Ways to Attract New,
Well-Pay Clients
Become Your Own Life Coach in 12 Easy Steps
How to Motivate Yourself
Online Marketing for Non-Techies: Turn Your
Website into a Sales Machine
One Day She Woke Up and Realized She Was Brave
She Said She Would Be Rich and They Believed
Her

I offer telephone coaching.
Contact me to set up an appointment!

growpublications@yahoo.com

**Learn more about Dr. Lyn and becoming a
Certified Professional Coach (CPC) at
http://www.growtraininginstitute.com/**

Follow me on
Facebook: http://facebook.com/ lyn.kelley1
Twitter: http://wefollow.com/JanesGoodAdvice
LinkedIn: http://www.linkedin.com/in/drlynisin

Thank You!

www.ingramcontent.com/pod-product-compliance
Lightning Source LLC
Chambersburg PA
CBHW071213260726
48653CB00041B/476